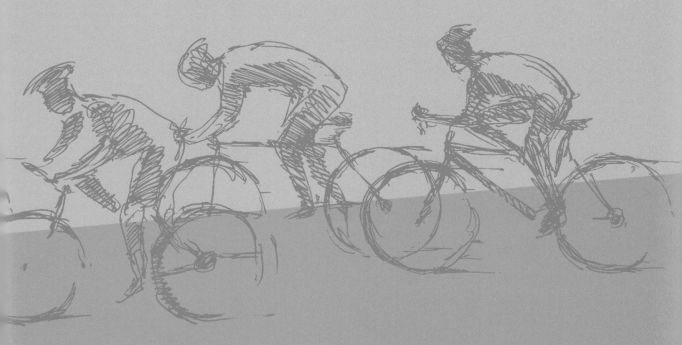

the
cyclingchef
on the go

BLOOMSBURY SPORT
Bloomsbury Publishing Plc
50 Bedford Square, London, WC1B 3DP, UK
29 Earlsfort Terrace, Dublin 2, Ireland

BLOOMSBURY, BLOOMSBURY SPORT and the Diana logo are trademarks of Bloomsbury Publishing Plc

First published in Great Britain 2024

Copyright © Alan Murchison, 2024
Food photography © Clare Winfield
Lifestyle photography © Daniel Gould
Design by Emil Dacanay and Sian Rance for D.R. Ink
Cycling photography © Getty Images

A catalogue record for this book is available from the British Library

Library of Congress Cataloguing-in-Publication data has been applied for

ISBN: HB: 978-1-3994-1106-6; ePUB: 978-1-3994-1105-9; EPDF: 978-1-3994-1108-0

2 4 6 8 10 9 7 5 3 1

Typeset in Miller Display
Printed and bound in China by C&C Offset Printing Co., Ltd.

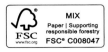

To find out more about our authors and books visit www.bloomsbury.com and sign up for our newsletters

the cyclingchef
on the go

Ride Day Recipes to Fuel Up, Replenish and Restore

ALAN MURCHISON

BLOOMSBURY SPORT

LONDON · OXFORD · NEW YORK · NEW DELHI · SYDNEY

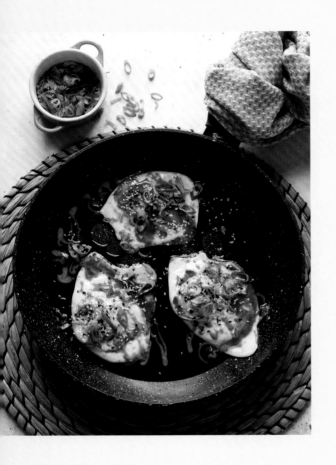

RECIPES

BACK-POCKET HEROES

CARBS ARE KING

PROTEIN PUNCHEURS

POST- AND PRE-RIDE EATS AND TREATS

WORKING UP A THIRST

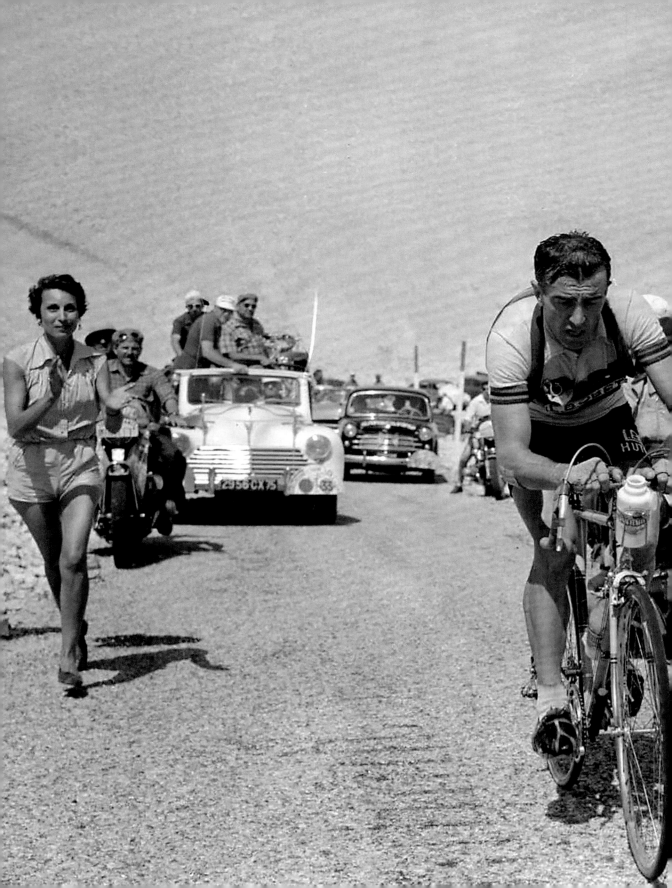

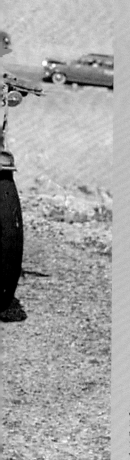

INTRODUCTION

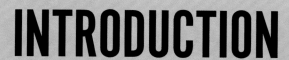

If you're hungry, it's too late. That's the cyclist's mantra. No one wants to run out of energy and hit the wall, so to professional, club and weekend riders alike, portable foods are as essential as a pump and a spare tube. Appetising on-the-bike snacks that enable you to refuel as you pedal are the key to enjoying that perfect ride, whether it's a race, a training run or a trip out with your mates on a sunny day.

Louison Bobet is cheered on by his wife as he climbs Mont Ventoux on his way to winning the 11th stage in 1955. Following this win, he went on to claim his third consecutive Tour de France.

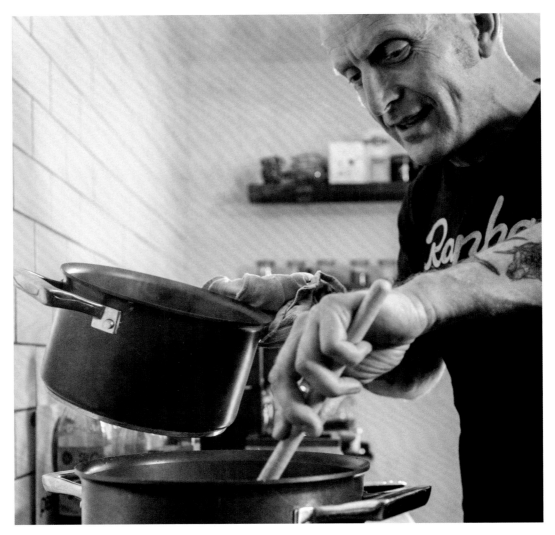

Preparing your own snacks and meals means you know exactly what is going into the food you'll consume. Using recognisable ingredients, you can prepare nutritionally targeted dishes for pre- and post-ride meals and on-the-bike snacks.

On-the-go food has to have certain qualities, though. It must be appealing enough to encourage snacking when appetites are blunted and robust enough to withstand being grabbed from your back pocket. It needs to moisten your dry mouth, but not leave your fingers sticky, and it must provide just the right amount of nutrients. The energy-boosting recipes in these pages provide portable snacks and drinks that fit the bill perfectly, leaving you to get on with catching the break, getting up that hill or going full gas in the final sprint.

Of course, fuelling doesn't start and end with what you consume on the bike. Other sections of this book provide easily prepared recipes for time-poor riders who have busy lives as well as a bike that needs riding. They include pre-ride breakfasts and drinks to make sure you begin your ride fully fuelled, as well as great tasting, fill-the-tank meals to help you recover after a gruelling session, or just a pleasantly tiring day in the saddle, without raiding the fridge or ordering a delivery.

These recipes are based around dishes I have created as a performance chef to leading teams and elite riders around the world. They are designed to deliver slow-releasing carbs, raise plunging energy levels, and to provide protein for aching muscles, and nutrients and electrolytes for healthy organs. Some I've developed to stave off those hunger pangs in the long hours out on the road; others will keep you going right to the finish line; and a few are for those times when home is a long way away and you just need cheering up!

You'll find all the recipes included here are easy and quick to make, and suitable for an athlete's diet plan. There are variations on old favourites, like the Ham, Parmesan and feta rice cakes; homages to cycling greats, such as Cheeky chicken Dowsett style; sweet treats like the Last legs espresso brownies; and more than the odd surprise, such as the Miso Marmite pancakes.

I hope the recipes in this book will encourage you to ditch those processed energy bars, sugary drinks and takeaways, and enjoy real food, full of flavour, that will prepare you for, see you through and help you get over even the toughest ride.

Eat well, ride well.
Alan Murchison

> **The energy-boosting recipes in these pages provide portable snacks and drinks that fit the bill perfectly, leaving you to get on with catching the break, getting up that hill or going full gas in the final sprint.**

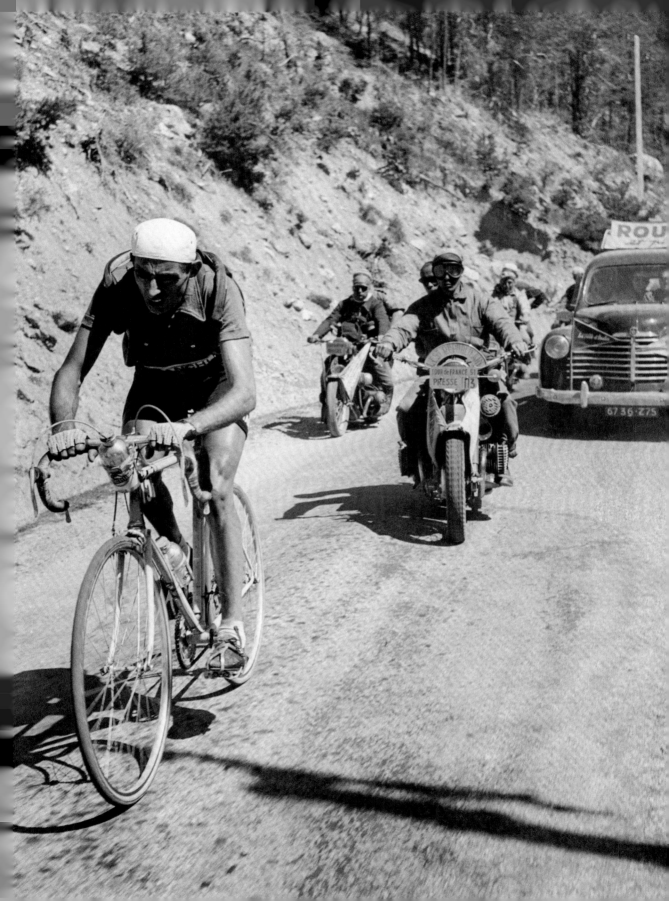

PREPARATION IS EVERYTHING

You're getting ready for a long day's ride. You check the weather forecast before you go. Is it a tights, rain jacket and overshoes day? How many layers do you need? That's all excellent preparation, but when it comes to food, you just grab a banana, a 'healthy' fruit and nut bar and maybe a gel, just in case. However, fuel management is just as important as your clothing and time spent planning your on-the-bike sustenance will not be wasted.

Italian legend Fausto Coppi rides the 1951 Tour de France. Coppi was still grieving after the death of his brother who died in his arms in a race accident just weeks earlier. Coppi finished the tour in 10th place overall as Hugo Koblet rode to a surprise victory.

Planning should focus on the intensity and duration of the ride. Will you be going full gas all day or just at certain points in the ride? How challenging are the climbs or is there a long, draining stretch?

The chances are you won't have a support vehicle driving by to hand you fresh water or feeding stations distributing provisions, so pay attention to how you pack your musette or fill your pockets and be aware of your route. Note the shops and petrol stations you'll be passing where you can replenish supplies.

The Spring Classic pro races or the Monuments are useful reference points. While the Grand Tour stage races generally allow plenty of opportunities for riders to approach team cars, receive food from domestiques or grab something from a roadside soigneur, the one-day races have few such luxuries. Narrow roads often restrict access by team cars and the constant intensity of racing full gas all day in godawful weather makes feeding difficult. When you're negotiating a cobbled section that requires maximum attention it's madness to reach into your pocket to grab a snack, however much you may need it. In these races, the riders' intake is carefully planned. They know what they will need and exactly when they will consume it. In fact, you'll often see a feeding schedule pasted to their stem.

Planning should focus on the intensity and duration of the ride. Will you be going full gas all day or just at certain points in the ride? How challenging are the climbs or is there a long, draining stretch? When are the key times you'll need to boost your energy levels? These types of questions should help you judge where and with what you choose to refuel.

SOURCING ENERGY

During low- to medium-intensity exercise, most of the energy you use is sourced from fats. Most club cyclists will carry about 10 per cent body fat and, as 500 g of fat stores just under 4000 calories, there is little to worry about. However, when the going gets tough, it's a different story. Muscles want energy and they want it NOW, so they'll turn to your glycogen stores, which will empty out after around 2000 calories max. During exercise, glycogen synthesis more or less slows to a halt and with no more stored glycogen your muscles immediately commandeer any carbs you consume to use as fuel.

It's a pretty rapid process. The intestine absorbs the carbs and breaks them down into sugars, which are delivered to the muscles. This can take as little as 10 minutes and most people's stomachs are capable of absorbing around 60 g of carbohydrates as a baseline. However, with some gut training this can fairly easily be taken up to 120 g an hour. Half a flapjack (as in 50 g) has 22 g of carbs. As a general rule, a 50 g bar or energy ball has 20 g of carbs and a banana has 20 g of carbs. It's worth noting that 100 g of Haribo has 80 g of carbs, which can be a welcome alternative to bars or gels. But here's the twist: all sugars are equal, but some are more equal than others. There is glucose, the sugar you'll find in most of the goodies in your musette: baked goods, breads, chocolate, dried fruit, even potatoes. It's absorbed easily by the intestine and is used directly by the muscles as energy, so it's perfect for a decent, hard ride. Then there's fructose, which is naturally found in honey, berries and especially dried fruits. It, too, is absorbed quickly, but before it can be used it has to be converted to lactate and it's absorbed at only 30 g per hour, rather than the 60 g per hour for glucose. No contest?

For many riders whose exertions operate at well under the 60 g absorption rate, it is not an issue. A fruit juice, some dried apricots or a handful of raisins offer variety and energy. However, for those 'enjoying' a long, hard day in the saddle, fructose really comes into its own. The intestine has different mechanisms to absorb glucose and fructose, and they can work at the same time. By

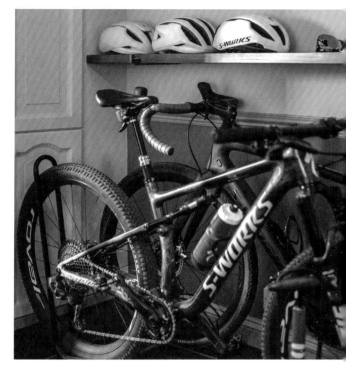

How many bikes does a cyclist need? Many swear by the n+1 rule, where n is the number of bikes currently owned.

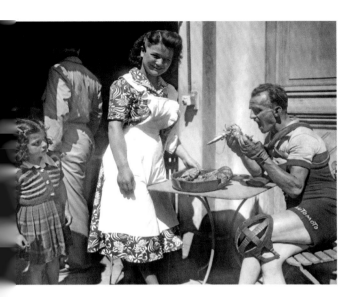

Food and drink to maintain energy levels on a ride can be sourced in different ways. You can carry energy-boosting snacks and drinks with you, have friends or support vehicles keeping you supplied from the roadside, or even, given time, nip into a cafe along the route.

balancing your sugar intake you can 'cheat' the system. A 2:1 glucose/fructose ratio can increase the absorption rate, with many duel-fuel drinks and gels providing a 1:0.8 ratio that, they claim, enables riders to increase their sugar absorption rate to 90 g an hour or more.

Once, elite riders were assumed to have the same 60–70g rate as mere mortals, but modern science continues to make advances. Around five years ago, a rate of 1g of carbohydrate per kg of bodyweight per hour (around 75 g for elite riders) was seen as viable. Chris Froome's legendary stage 19 victory in the 2018 Giro d'Italia with a solo break over the Colle delle Finestre saw him averaging around 100 g an hour throughout the five-hour stage. Since then, some pro riders have achieved levels of 120 g an hour. The change has come through a combination of scientific advances in gels and fuel drinks, and a focus on training the gut by gradually increasing the carb intake over the course of pre-season training.

Endurance athletes are especially prone to gastrointestinal (GI) problems and can suffer anything from constipation and bloating through to diarrhoea and vomiting. It's not a pleasant subject for a recipe book, but, hey, if it's going to feature anywhere it's in a book called *On the Go*. Anyone who remembers Tom Dumoulin losing two minutes when stomach cramps forced him to stop and defecate by the side of the road after climbing the Stelvio on stage 16 of the 2017 Giro d'Italia, will understand how devastating and costly, not to mention embarrassing, GI issues can be.

The main problem athletes face is how long it takes for the food and drink they've consumed to pass from the stomach to the intestine. This is called the gastric emptying rate. Unless the stomach empties, no absorption of sugars can take place, and this rate may be affected by stress, which can be driven by adrenaline and nerves, and the body may go into fight or flight mode. It is also a natural reaction to the body undergoing high-intensity activity. In addition, during strenuous exercise, the demand for blood from the muscles and the skin takes priority, and the subsequent reduction in blood flowing to the stomach limits its ability to function fully.

Easing up on the pedals is not an option, but there are steps you can take to alleviate the issues, with ensuring you're hydrated at all times being the most important. How well the stomach and the intestine function depends on, and is eased by, the presence of liquid. Other measures you should take are ensuring you keep as cool as possible, avoiding foods with a high-calorie density (having a lot of calories in a small quantity of food) or those that are very high in fibre, and eating regular, bite-sized portions.

TRAINING THE GUT

If that all sounds rather worrying, let me reassure you that the digestive system is a pretty good student. Training the gut is totally possible. Repeated experience can help it learn to take the strain of high-intensity, long-distance rides. Use your training to slowly increase your carb intake and your capacity to eat at regular intervals, and learn to drink water, more water and then more water again.

The key to it all is thinking about exactly what you're consuming, whether it's the off-season or you're training, racing or resting. Off the bike there is no substitute for a good, balanced diet of real food that provides for a healthy gut, while preparation and an understanding of fuelling your ride correctly can make a massive difference to your riding experience and your times.

CARBO RINSING

Swishing a liquid around your mouth and spitting it out is probably something you're more used to doing at the dentist than on a bike, but it might be worth giving it a try. Carbo rinsing has gained significant scientific backing over the past few years with some studies confirming that just flushing a carbohydrate-based drink around your mouth for around 10 seconds can improve performance levels.

A sports drink, watered down fruit juice or even sugared water have all given positive effects in research, when the rinsing is performed at regular five- to ten-minute intervals over a period of around an hour. Taste receptors sensitive to carbohydrates send messages to the brain, which, fooled into thinking food is coming, boosts mood and energy levels. If it works, it can be useful for anyone on a low-carb training programme or those who don't want to consume carbs at the end of a ride.

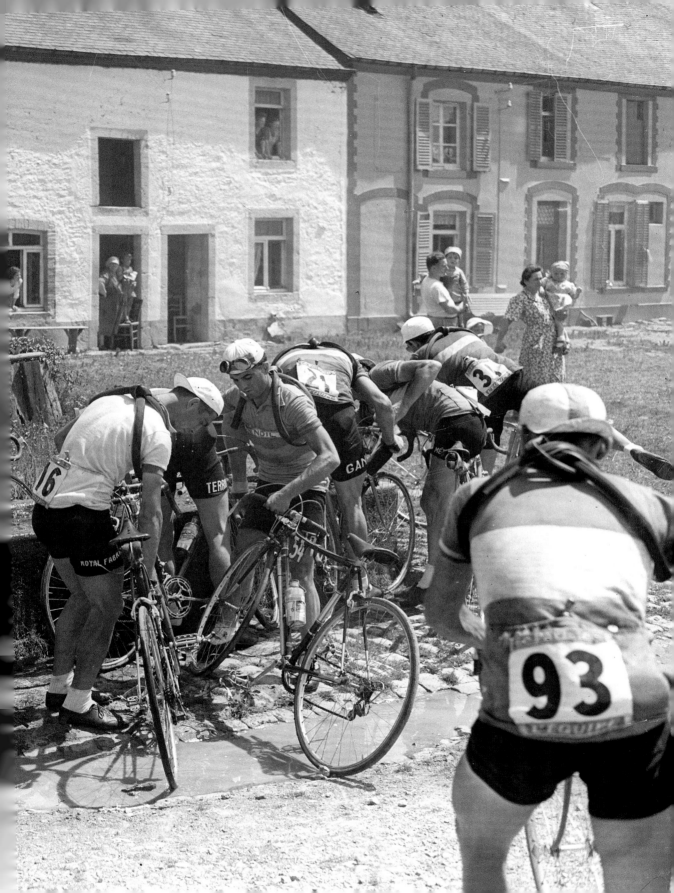

FUEL FOR PERFORMANCE

Let me get it straight out there: up to 90 per cent of riders – casual, club or pro – don't eat enough on the bike. Yes, you heard me right. Fuelling correctly is just as essential as having your saddle set at the right height or wearing the right shoes, and failing to prepare and pay attention to your blood sugar levels is a recipe for disaster on any ride requiring notable effort.

Tour de France riders stop to fill up their bidons. Staying hydrated and keeping well fuelled is the best way to avoid the dreaded bonk – that cyclist's nightmare when energy levels start to rapidly drain away.

For maximum performance, your food and drink intake should be planned according to the intensity and duration of the ride.

Food as fuel is not a reward or a treat. It is not a cream cake mid-point through a ride or a Big Mac and fries when you finish. For maximum performance, your food and drink intake should be planned according to the intensity and duration of the ride. That isn't to say it should not be flavoursome or tasty, though, because the more appealing a snack, the less likely you are to postpone or skip eating it.

Riders' diets require a mix of macronutrients (nutrients required in high quantities): protein for muscle repair, fat for low intensity exercise and organ protection, and carbohydrates for energy. Polyunsaturated fats should make up around 20 per cent to 25 per cent of your diet, but the relative percentages and quantities of the other two can vary considerably depending on the frequency and rigour of the riding you're doing.

Carbohydrate is pure fuel. The body breaks down carbohydrates into glucose, which is the main source of energy for the body's cells, tissues and organs. It can be used immediately or stored in the liver and muscles as glycogen. However, there is a limit to the amount of glycogen the body can retain. It varies from person to person, but it's around 500 g. That equates to just 60 to 90 minutes of strenuous exercise. Pure and simple, this is the reason we need to continually refuel when out on a hard ride of more than an hour in duration.

Pre-ride carbo-loading is therefore key. Your glycogen levels need to be topped up before you begin your ride. Depending on the length of your ride, you may not need to carbo-load on the evening before an event and a normal balanced meal will often suffice. However, a more testing day might call for a carbohydrate-heavy breakfast or pre-race meal a couple of hours before the start to fill up the tank.

THE BONK

A car doesn't care how it gets petrol, whether it's from the pump, a can or an old lemonade bottle, and your body isn't fussy about where it gets its carbs from. If you're on a long drive you'll eventually end up pulling into the petrol station again, but tucking into a bowl of pasta after 40k of your sportive isn't an option, so regular refills are essential. You might not be hungry at all. You might not feel like anything sweet. You may be knackered and eating something is the last thing you can be bothered with. Or maybe you're just too engrossed in the actual riding to even think about food. Wrong, wrong, wrong. Your performance will gradually suffer as your energy depletes and you could be on the road to the nightmare zone they call the bonk.

It's officially called hypoglycaemia, where the level of glucose in your blood drops so low that it affects your normal functioning. Cyclists nickname it the bonk or refer to hitting the wall and few haven't been ambushed by it at some point in their riding lives – often more than once. Your body and mind are pretty adept at hiding the symptoms, and it's a sneaky bastard that creeps up on you. Adrenalin, which kicks in whenever the body is under stress, masks the effects of falling blood sugar and your own denial does the rest.

You might struggle to do your pull at the front, lose contact with the back marker or find the climb tougher than you expected. At this point you should reduce your effort so your body reverts to burning fat and eat something sharpish. I say should, but so often you don't, because you tell yourself there are lots of possible reasons you're finding it difficult: you're not working hard enough; yes, you're a bit tired, but you can ride through it; or it's just the end of a race, a long ride or a challenging climb, so of course you're weary.

You may not even notice there's a problem, but woolly thinking isn't a coincidence. It's not just the legs burning through the glucose reserves. The brain relies on supplies of glucose, too. As levels drop, so does your brain power. Your decision-making can suffer and, as you start to lose control of your emotions, you might become angry, confused and even depressed. It is now too late to ease up, take a snack and go again. The French sometimes call the condition *l'homme au marteau* – the man with the hammer – and he is waiting for you just up the road.

Once all your glucose is being diverted to your brain, you are done for (and that's saying it politely). Your body is overwhelmed by fatigue, your legs feel like jelly and you can barely turn the pedals. You feel light-headed, even faint, and you're possibly nauseous or suffering from blurred vision. All you can do is the supermarket raid. Anywhere that sells chocolate and coke. Get plenty of it and sit by the side of the road munching and guzzling. When you've finished feeling sorry for yourself, you'll remember turning down that half a brownie your mate offered you an hour ago and you'll probably feel a bit stupid.

So, you ask, how often and how much do I have to eat on the road? The evasive but honest answer is that it can vary wildly. It depends on the duration and intensity of the race, and even then different individuals react differently to glucose and the stress that exercise puts their bodies under. Blood sugar spikes last longer for some than others, while there are riders who find that eating carbs

THE RED AMBULANCE

Nutritionists will tell you there is absolutely nothing healthy about Coca-Cola, but that doesn't stop plenty of cyclists regularly downing the black gold – and that includes a fair number of professionals. In fact, Ed Clancy swears he's won three gold medals on the stuff, but there is a time and a place for everything.

The place is when the end of the ride is in sight; the time is when your energy levels have gone into the red and the danger lights are flashing. That's when you call for the red ambulance. A can of Coke will give you a slight caffeine hit (35 mg), which is just enough to bring a little focus to a fuzzy mind. The bubbles can help soothe a fatigued, upset stomach and a whack of sugar (39 g) should raise your energy levels enough to get you to the finish line.

Just as importantly, there's something comforting about that familiar red can that's a real morale boost when you're up against it. There's a shack at the top of one of the popular training climbs in Majorca. The guy there sells cans of coke to exhausted cyclists at four Euros a pop – talk about a licence to print money!

before protein and fat, or vice versa, can affect the stability of their energy levels.

One approach is to use your training rides to assess how your body responds to different quantities and sources of glucose. These days, many pro riders train with glucose monitors. These use a small sensor stuck to the skin which tracks and relays real-time glucose levels to a wrist display. The fact that UCI currently ban these in races shows just how much of an advantage it is to keep a check on the level of your energy reserves. Some may find the current high price restrictive, but hiring one for a short training period is a realistic option. There is no doubt that they will soon be in widespread use.

A more practical answer is to do something every 20 minutes after the first hour of riding, whether that's taking a gulp of water or eating a piece of banana or a rice cake. Put an alarm on to remind yourself if necessary. Feeding yourself regular, small amounts during the ride will also help your post-ride recovery. Come home with a calorie deficit and you are likely to lay waste to the contents of the fridge. You'll feel nauseous, bloated and will blow a hole in any weight control plan you have. Any cake, crisps or chocolate you devour now are not going to help you in the present and any calories that do need to be replaced can be done over the next few hours. Eat for performance not for reward. Food is one of life's greatest pleasures, but rewarding yourself after exercise should be an occasional luxury not a habitual practice.

These fuelling principles apply to anyone out riding seriously for over an hour, but exactly how much you need to consume is personal. This is particularly true for women, because fluctuations in hormone levels during the menstrual cycle can have a significant effect on how your metabolism works at any given time. Use your training sessions to monitor and experiment with your consumption in coordination with a power meter.

JUST ENOUGH

There's only one thing worse than not eating enough on the bike and that's eating too much. Overeating can affect your performance. As I explained on page 15, your stomach can only process 60 g of carbohydrates at any one time so, unless you've been specifically training to increase your consumption, any more than this and the food will sit in your gut, quite possibly causing indigestion, bloating, nausea or excessive gas.

The answer is to be realistic about your fuelling requirements. If your glycogen levels are topped up and a large section of the ride is at a moderate pace, you may need to consume far less than you think. Use trial and error to get to know how much your body needs and work on the basis of taking in 'just enough'. Learn to recognise the fluctuations in energy levels. Keep your portions very small and top up with extra when necessary. Around 20 g of carbohydrate can restore your glycogen levels in 10 minutes or so.

That's good advice for normal folk, but some pro teams are turning just-enough eating into a precise science. Data researcher Kristian van Kuijk has developed algorithms to calculate riders' required calorie intakes, taking into consideration not just an individual cyclist's BMI, but also variables such as weather conditions or race tactics. It might be a while before this approach is open to the rest of us, but then the tech is constantly changing, so don't quote me on that.

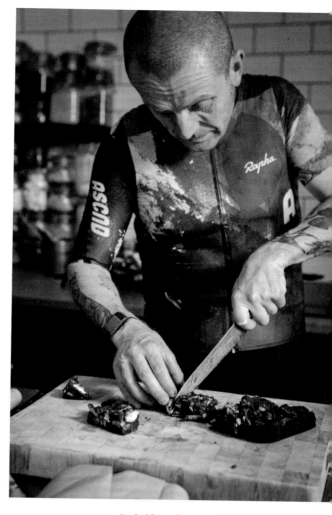

On-the-bike snacks need to fit neatly into your back pocket, be easy to handle and provide the right amount of nutrition when needed. You don't need a ruler for precision cutting (unless that's how you roll); just divide your snacks into roughly equal bite-sized pieces.

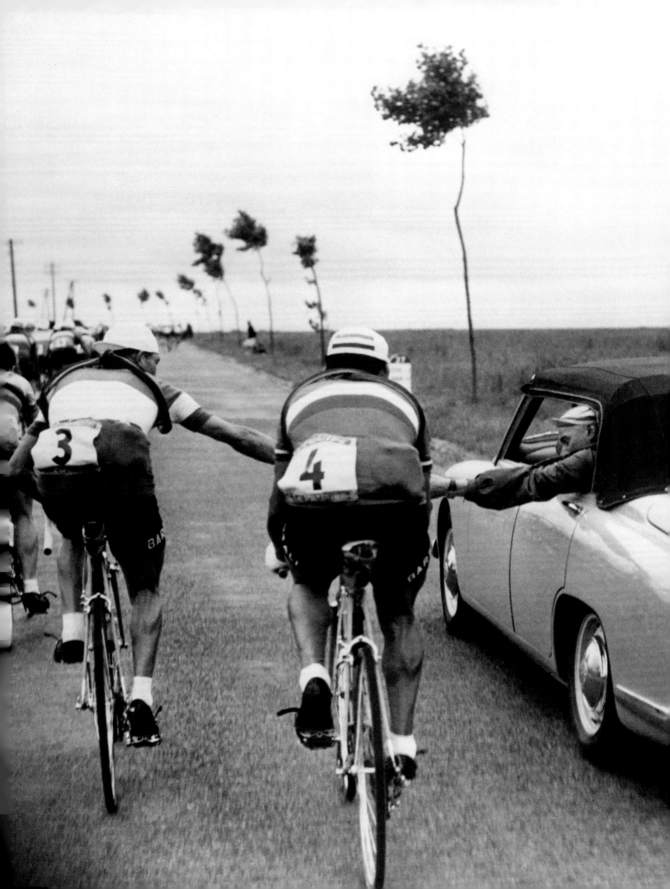

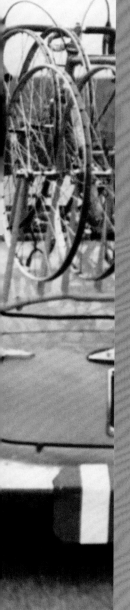

RECIPES
BACK-POCKET HEROES

It could be a Spectacular speculoos rice cake (see page 55), a Tortilla-wrapped sushi roll (see page 56) or a Snickerish slice (see page 36), but whatever you pull out of that back pocket when you're on the bike has a job to do. Yes, it has to deliver an energy boost – and these pick-me-ups are guaranteed to lift you mid-ride – but it also has to deliver an exciting flavour and texture profile. These recipes have been developed to do just that.

The great Gino Bartali (3) riding the flat routes of Normandy on the fifth stage of the 1953 Tour de France. At 39, the Italian's career was coming to a close, but he had already won two Tours and remains the only rider to win three consecutive mountain stages in the race.

BÄCKSTEDT BARS

A high-carb, low-fibre, energy blast inspired by the amazing world class racer Zoe Bäckstedt and ideal for any rider with a busy life.

This is a sweet treat you can tuck into any time, especially when you're on the move and snacking in challenging locations, so it's perfect for those chillier conditions… like a filthy cold Belgian cyclo-cross race!

Makes 12

125 g (4 oz) Coco Pops

1 tablespoon cocoa powder

pinch of sea salt flakes

25 g (1 oz) unsalted butter

50 g (2 oz) golden syrup

40 g ($1\frac{1}{2}$ oz) 70 per cent chocolate

100 g ($3\frac{1}{2}$ oz) white marshmallows

Nutrition per serving:
Energy: 119 kcal | Total carbohydrate: 20 g (of which sugars: 13 g)
Fat: 3.6 g | Fibre: 0.7 g | Protein: 1.4 g | Salt: 0.2 g

1. Line a 20 x 20 cm (8 x 8 in) tray or loaf tin with greaseproof paper.

2. Mix the Coco Pops, cocoa powder and salt together and set aside.

3. Melt the butter and syrup together, add the chocolate and stir well.

4. Add the marshmallows to the chocolatey mix and melt over a low heat.

5. Stir the chocolatey marshmallow mix into the Coco Pops mix.

6. Pour into the lined tray or lined loaf tin and refrigerate for 90 minutes.

7. Cut into decent-size chunks and store in the fridge. They'll last forever… except they won't!

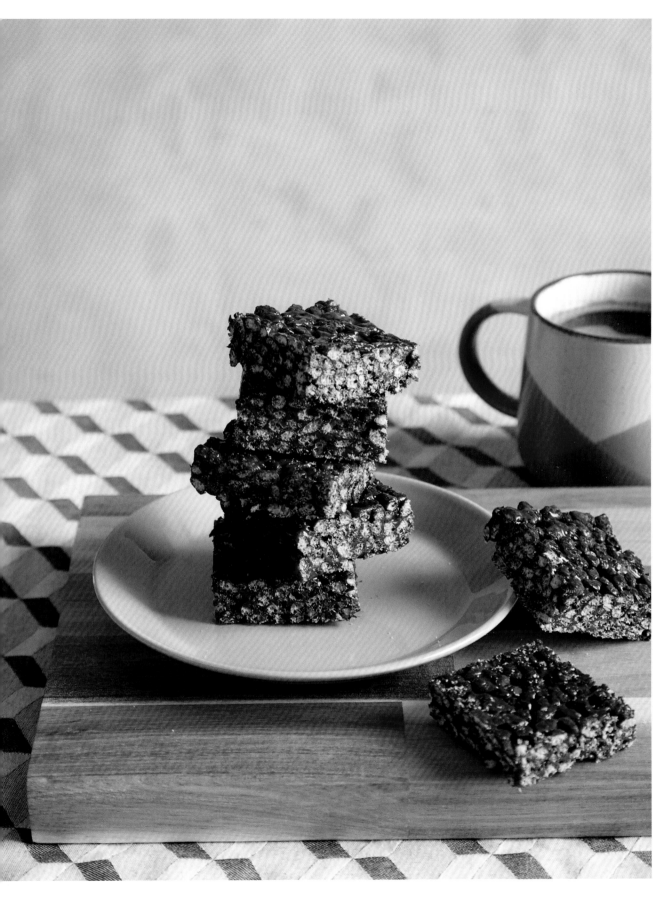

FLUFFY CARROT CAKE WAFFLES

These are a variation on a renowned cycling favourite and they are equally good as a before-you-go breakfast as on-the-bike food.

If you don't have a waffle-maker, a toasted sandwich-maker will work fine or, failing that, a pan, but make plenty of batter as it sits really well in the fridge for a couple of days.

Serves 6

75 g (3 oz) butter

200 g (7 oz) grated carrot

80 g (3 oz) maple syrup

2 teaspoons ground cassia cinnamon bark

1 teaspoon allspice

freshly ground black pepper

Batter

2 large eggs

500 ml (2 cups) unsweetened almond milk

100 g ($3\frac{1}{2}$ oz) butter, melted

1 teaspoon vanilla extract

1 teaspoon freshly grated nutmeg

450 g (1 lb) self-raising flour

Nutrition per serving:

Energy: 449 kcal | Total carbohydrate: 66g (of which sugars: 11 g)

Fat: 14 g | Fibre: 4.8 g | Protein: 11 g | Salt: 0.85 g

1. Melt the butter in a sauté pan. Cook the grated carrot in the butter over a medium heat for 3–4 minutes. Add the maple syrup and spices, cook down until sticky, set aside and allow to cool.

2. Separate the eggs. Whisk together the egg yolks, milk, melted butter, vanilla and nutmeg. Gradually whisk in the flour until you have a smooth batter, then stir in the carrot mix.

3. Whisk the egg whites until they form soft peaks. Take one-third of the egg whites and add the batter. Stir well, then fold through the remaining two-thirds of the egg whites, trying to retain as much air as you can.

4. Preheat your waffle-maker, then cook each waffle for 4–6 minutes, or 2–3 minutes each side if slumming it in a non-stick pan.

5. If cooking for friends, keep the waffles warm in the oven at a low heat. These can be made in advance and reheated.

PARSNIP CHOC CHIP COCONUT WAFFLES

The waffle-maker has brought a whole new dimension to the cyclist-friendly snack.

These simple-to-make, denser-than-usual waffles are robust enough to survive a trip in the back pocket, too, and the nutty parsnip is a perfect partner for the coconut and chocolate, plus this recipe requires no fancy egg-whipping.

Serves 6

225 g (8 oz) self-raising flour

60 g (2½ oz) desiccated coconut

80 g (3 oz) grated parsnip

1 tablespoon creamed coconut

1 medium egg

275 ml (1 cup) light coconut milk

50 g (2 oz) coconut oil, melted

60 g (2½ oz) 70 per cent choc chips

Nutrition per serving:
Energy: 401kcal | Total carbohydrate: 34 g (of which sugars: 4.9g)
Fat: 25 g | Fibre: 5.5 g | Protein: 7.1 g | Salt: 0.38 g

1. Mix the dry ingredients – the self-raising flour, desiccated coconut and grated parsnip – together.

2. Place the dry mix into the bowl of a mixer and use the paddle attachment to incorporate the creamed coconut, egg, coconut milk and coconut oil. If it seems too dry, add an extra small splash of coconut milk.

3. At the last minute, stir in the choc chips.

4. Preheat your waffle-maker, then cook each waffle for 4–6 minutes or 2–3 minutes each side if slumming it in a non-stick pan.

5. If cooking for friends, keep the waffles warm in the oven at a low heat. These can be made in advance and reheated.

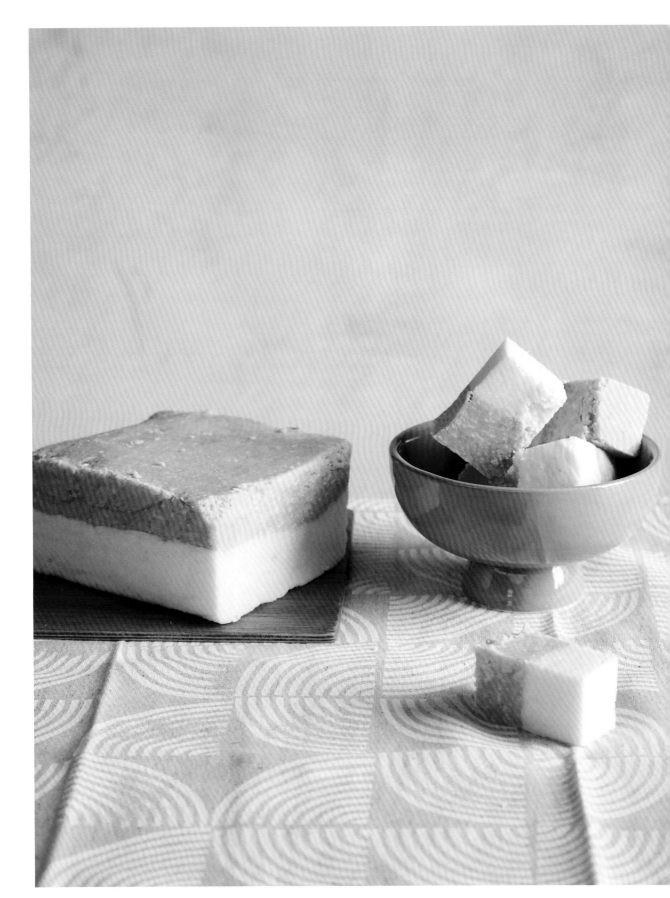

RETROTASTIC COCONUT ICE

Step back in time with this pure and simple energy hit using only three ingredients.

Revived and tested especially for those youngsters who have never been exposed to condensed milk with added sugar! Totally retro, but a life saver when the legs are empty, coconut ice is best eaten while wearing a woollen cycling jersey and chatting about Eddy Merckx, as that is also retrotastic!

Makes 24

1 tin (397 g/14 oz) sweetened condensed milk

450 g (1 lb) icing sugar, sieved

350 g (12 oz) desiccated coconut

red food colouring

2 teaspoons chocolate chips (optional)

Nutrition per serving:

Energy: 222 kcal | Total carbohydrate: 29 g (of which sugars: 28 g)

Fat: 10 g | Fibre: 3.1 g | Protein: 2.2 g | Salt: 0.05 g

1. Place the condensed milk in the bowl of a food processor. Gradually add the icing sugar and mix.

2. Next add the coconut until it forms a firm paste. If the mix is too wet, add a little more coconut. For the full retro effect, split the mix into two and add a splash of red food colouring to one half to make half the mix pink!

3. Line a 24 x 12 cm (2 lb) loaf tin. Add half the mix to the tin – let's go white first – and press it down firmly and evenly. Refrigerate for an hour. Then layer the pink mix on top, adding the chocolate chips if using, and refrigerate again to set. When nice and firm, cut into pink and white chunks.

4. Alternatively, divide the mix into two, roll each half into a long thick sausage, wrap in cling film and when firm cut into discs.

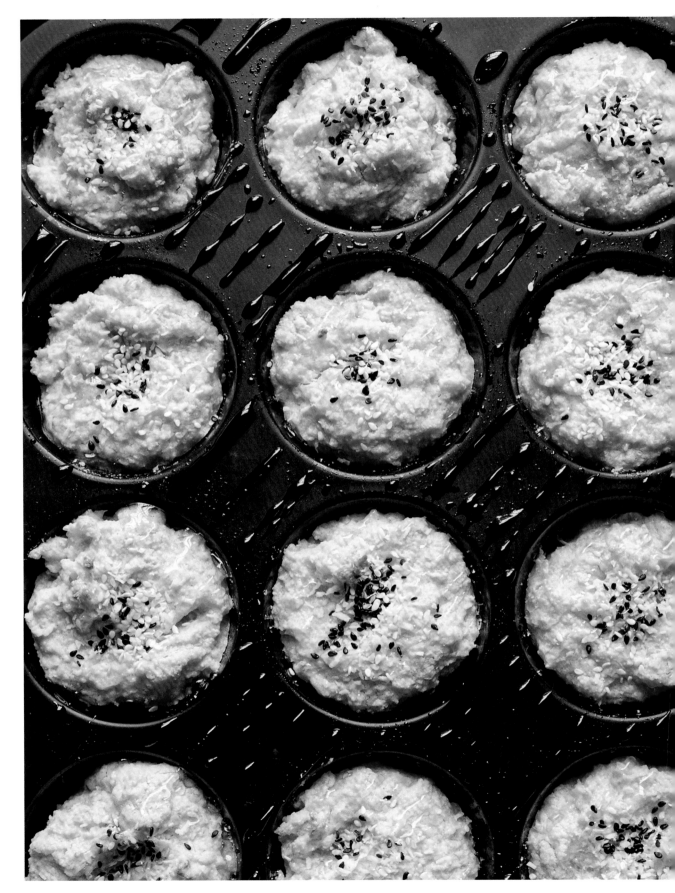

MURCH MOCHI JAPANESE-STYLE CORN AND COCONUT CAKE

Looking for a high-energy hit that isn't too sweet?

Super-soft, deliciously chewy and a little different, these Far East-inspired rice cakes have fantastic flavour and texture. Based on Japanese mochi – sticky rice balls – all the ingredients are blended into one batter, packing a whole lot of nutrients into one cake.

Makes 12

200 g (7 oz) sushi rice

1 teaspoon turmeric

1 teaspoon baking powder

260 g (9 $\frac{1}{4}$ oz) tinned sweetcorn

200 g (7 oz) coconut cream

2 medium eggs

125 g (4 oz) coconut oil

1 teaspoon vanilla extract

40 g (1$\frac{1}{2}$ oz) toasted coconut

1 teaspoon black sesame seeds

Nutrition per serving:
Energy: 321 kcal | Total carbohydrate: 17 g (of which sugars: 2.9 g)
Fat: 26 g | Fibre: 1.6 g | Protein: 4.2 g | Salt: 0.15 g

1. Preheat the oven to 180°C/350°F/Gas 4 and grease a silicon 12-cup cake tray.

2. Grind the sushi rice in a food processor until it's a fine powder. If that isn't possible, then use rice flour.

3. Add the turmeric and baking powder, and mix well.

4. Next throw in the sweetcorn, coconut cream, eggs and coconut oil, and blend until you have a fine paste.

5. Then add the vanilla extract and 90 per cent of the toasted coconut, keeping some back for the topping.

6. Press the mixture into the cake tray moulds and top with some toasted coconut and the black sesame seeds.

7. Bake for 20–22 minutes. Allow to cool and then store at room temperature for up to two days. They can be kept in the fridge, but it's better not to eat them chilled.

MAGHS' MAPLE BUTTER SABLE BISCUITS

French Canadian cyclo-cross star Maghalie Rochette introduced maple butter to me.

It was a culinary revelation and ideal for a take on a traditional French biscuit, so this is for Maghs – a biscuit that is more robust than shortbread and an ideal on-the-bike bite. Anyone who has had to scoop crumbs out of their back pocket will know why that's a big plus.

Makes 16

80 g (3 oz) Canadian maple butter

90 g ($3\frac{1}{2}$ oz) salted French butter

110 g ($3\frac{1}{2}$ oz) golden Demerara sugar

2 eggs yolks

1 pinch of salt

295 g ($10\frac{1}{2}$ oz) plain flour

1 whole egg

Nutrition per serving:
Energy: 176 kcal | Total carbohydrate: 22 g (of which sugars: 8.4 g)
Fat: 8.3 g | Fibre: 0.8 g | Protein: 2.9 g | Salt: 0.2 g

1. Place the maple butter, salted butter and sugar into the bowl of a mixer and use the paddle attachment to beat them for 3–4 minutes until light and creamy in texture.

2. Add the egg yolks and mix again.

3. Add the salt and gradually add the flour until well mixed, but do not overwork the dough.

4. Roll the dough into a ball and place it in the fridge for 30–45 minutes.

5. Preheat the oven to 180°C/350°F/Gas 4.

6. Roll out the dough on a flour-dusted worktop to a 5 mm ($\frac{1}{4}$ in) thickness. Cut into 5 cm (2 in) rounds and place on a non-stick baking sheet.

7. Prick the biscuits with a fork. Beat the whole egg and brush the top of the biscuits with it.

8. Bake the biscuits for 12–15 minutes until golden brown. Allow to cool and then place in an airtight container, where they will keep for three to four days.

BIGHAM'S GOLDEN BALLS

A carb hit and a moreish flavour was the brief.

The oats, raisins and honey came good and the pina colada vibe sealed the deal. In homage to former world hour record-holder Dan Bigham, these super-snacks are 'almost' guaranteed to give you 7 to 10 watts in gains.

Makes 16

100 g (3½ oz) golden raisins

150 ml (⅔ cup) pineapple juice

200 g (7 oz) rolled oats

50 g (2 oz) dried pineapple

100 g (3½ oz) honey

100 g (3½ oz) nut butter

50 g (2 oz) desiccated coconut

60 g (2½ oz) chopped glace cherries

pinch of ground ginger

pinch of salt

Nutrition per serving:
Energy: 172 kcal | Total carbohydrate: 24 g (of which sugars: 14 g)
Fat: 6.3 g | Fibre: 2.5 g | Protein: 3.6 g | Salt: 0.19 g

1. Simmer the raisins in the pineapple juice until the liquid reduces to a sticky glaze.

2. Blend the oats, sticky raisins and pineapple together in a food processor.

3. Add the honey and nut butter, and mix until it all comes together.

4. Then stir in the desiccated coconut, cherries, ginger and salt. If the mix is a little bit wet, add more coconut.

5. Roll into 16 balls – each one should weigh about 50 g (2 oz) – and dust with coconut again. These can be stored in the fridge for up to 2 weeks.

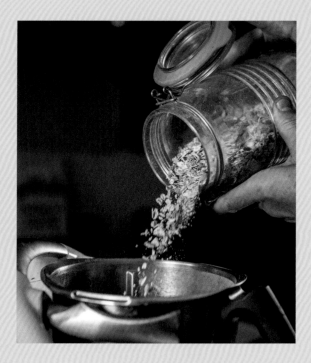

Don't scrimp on your herbs and spices. They not only add unique flavours, aromas and colour to the dishes, but they carry health benefits too, including antioxidant, anti-inflammatory and blood-sugar regulating properties.

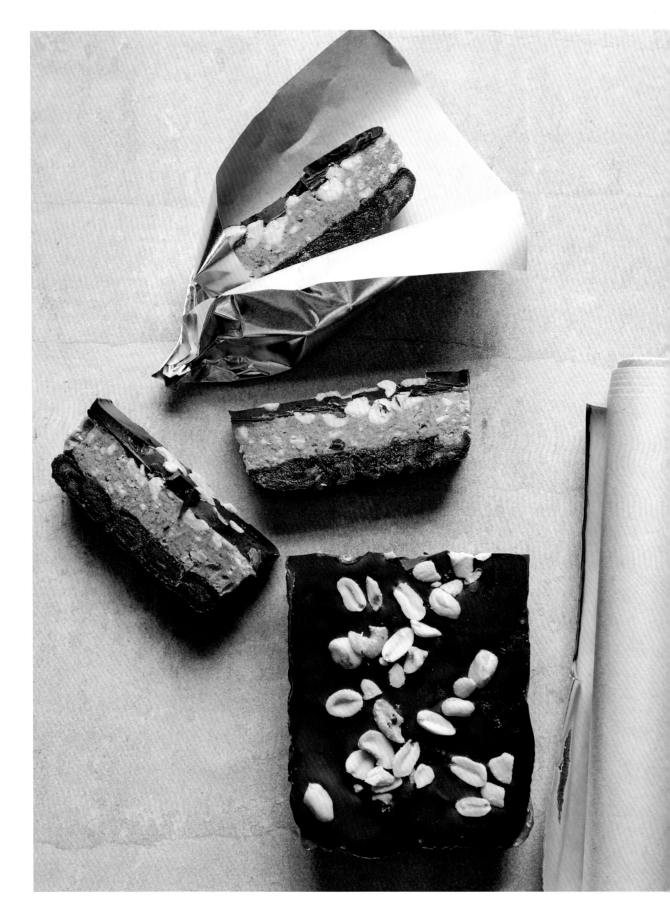

SNICKERISH SLICES

Time to play around with a classic flavour combo.

When mixed with nut butter and chocolate, the Medjool dates really taste like toffee, but a healthier toffee. These slices are good for post-ride snackage too, and great with a dollop of full fat Greek yoghurt.

Makes 16

16 large Medjool dates

75 g (3 oz) coconut oil

300 g (11 oz) nut butter

100 g ($3\frac{1}{2}$ oz) salted peanuts

100 g ($3\frac{1}{2}$ oz) 70 per cent chocolate

pinch of sea salt flakes

Nutrition per serving:
Energy: 316 kcal | Total carbohydrate: 22 g (of which sugars: 19 g)
Fat: 21 g | Fibre: 4.1 g | Protein: 8.2 g | Salt: 0.3 g

1. Line a 24 x 12 cm (2 lb) loaf tin with foil.

2. Remove the stones from the dates and place them in the bottom of the loaf tin. Ensure the base is fully covered and the dates are pressed down evenly. Refrigerate for 90 minutes.

3. Warm up the coconut oil and stir in the nut butter. Using a spatula, add this to the top of the dates and spread evenly.

4. Sprinkle on the salted peanuts, reserving a tablespoon of nuts for later, and refrigerate again to allow the nut butter to firm up.

5. Gently melt the chocolate, pour it over the nut butter layer, and sprinkle on the remaining nuts and a pinch of salt. Refrigerate once more to allow to set.

6. When cutting up, it's best to place it chocolate-side down on your chopping board. Store in the fridge in an airtight container.

BAKEWELL BALLS

Sometimes you can't beat an old favourite and the Bakewell tart has plenty of delicious flavour to satisfy your tastebuds.

However, it's a bit of a faff to make and a bit fragile for ride food, so here the almond and cherry tart taste appears in a cyclist-friendly bite-sized ball instead.

Makes 16

150 g (5 oz) rolled oats

100 g (3½ oz) ground almonds

180 g (6 oz) soft dates

2 teaspoons almond essence

150 g (5 oz) nut butter

50 g (2 oz) maple syrup

50 g (2 oz) chopped bitter dried cherries

50 g (2 oz) chopped glace cherries

150 g (5 oz) almond flakes

Nutrition per serving:
Energy: 259 kcal | Total carbohydrate: 22 g (of which sugars: 14 g)
Fat: 14 g | Fibre: 5 g | Protein: 7.5 g | Salt: 0.1 g

1. Blend the oats, ground almonds and dates in a food processor until the mix comes together.

2. Add the almond essence, nut butter and maple syrup. Blend until a large sticky ball forms.

3. Remove from the blender and use your hands to work in the chopped cherries and almond flakes.

4. Roll into small 50 g (2 oz) balls – if you're feeling cheffy you can roll the balls in almond nibs – and refrigerate. Store in the fridge.

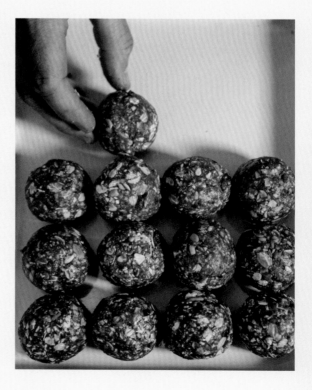

FRUIT 'N' NUTELLA BITES

Go to any pro bike race in the world and you'll find shaved legs, overweight ex-pros, very nice bikes, hungry riders and... Nutella!

It's like the best chocolatey fudge you will ever eat. There are just four ingredients here, plus optional extras, but your morale will go sky high when you dig one of these beauties out of your back pocket.

Makes 30

500 g (1 lb 2 oz) 60 per cent chocolate

420 g (15 oz) Nutella

200 g (7 oz) toasted whole hazelnuts

200 g (7 oz) raisins

75 g (3 oz) almond nibs (optional)

75 g (3 oz) cocoa nibs (optional)

Nutrition per serving (including toppings):
Energy: 274 kcal | Total carbohydrate: 21 g (of which sugars: 17 g)
Fat: 18 g | Fibre: 3.1 g | Protein: 4.5 g | Salt: 0.06 g

1. Line a 20 x 20 cm (8 x 8 in) tray or loaf tin with greaseproof paper.
2. Melt the chocolate in a bain-marie over a low heat.
3. Stir in the Nutella, hazelnuts and raisins.
4. Pour into the lined tray or loaf tin.
5. Sprinkle over optional almond and cocoa nibs if you fancy a crunchy topping.
6. Refrigerate for 2–3 hours then cut into bite-sized chunks. Store in the fridge for up to 2 weeks.

APRICOT, ALMOND AND FETA BITES

It's like a nutritional supergroup coming together – three stars of the cycling portables world on one snack-sized stage.

This simple sweet and savoury snack has great balance and texture, but not only does the apricot provide a superb energy boost, it acts as a neat holder for the feta and the nutrient-packed roasted almond.

Makes 12

12 soft dried apricots

120 g (4 oz) aged feta cheese

12 smoked roasted almonds

Nutrition per serving:
Energy: 52 kcal | Total carbohydrate: 3.7 g (of which sugars: 3.6 g)
Fat: 2.7 g | Fibre: 1.9 g | Protein: 2.2 g | Salt: 0.26 g

1. Open up the apricots to reveal a small pouch.
2. Cut the feta into 12 small cubes and stuff one into each apricot.
3. Repeat the process with the almonds.
4. Refrigerate for up to 24 hours. Wrap individually if you're taking them out on a ride.

JAFFA CAKEY CRUMPETS

Like crumpets? Like Jaffa Cakes? Then you'll just love these bitter orange and rich chocolate delights.

They're a breakfast or brunch treat to die for as the crumpet soaks up the orange marmalade like a sponge. Better still, they require almost zero cooking – just put them together and enjoy the flavour behaviour.

Makes 4

4 large crumpets

8 teaspoons Seville orange marmalade

4 teaspoons mixed candied peel/ caramelised orange

120 g (4 oz) 70 per cent chocolate

pinch of sea salt flakes

Nutrition per serving:
Energy: 311 kcal | Total carbohydrate: 40 g (of which sugars: 23 g)
Fat: 13 g | Fibre: 4.8g | Protein: 5.7g | Salt: 1.3g

1. Place the crumpets on a cooling rack with a tray underneath.

2. Spread the orange marmalade liberally on to the crumpets.

3. Top with most of the candied peel, reserving about 1 teaspoon.

4. Chop up and melt the chocolate, ensuring it doesn't get too hot. Allow it to cool a little and then spoon it over the marmalade-soaked crumpets in one thin layer.

5. Scatter a few chunks of the candied peel and some sea salt flakes on top of the melted chocolate.

6. Allow the crumpets to set in a cooler part of the kitchen, but don't refrigerate as the chocolate will set like a brick. Store in an airtight container and keep somewhere cool. Eat within two or three days.

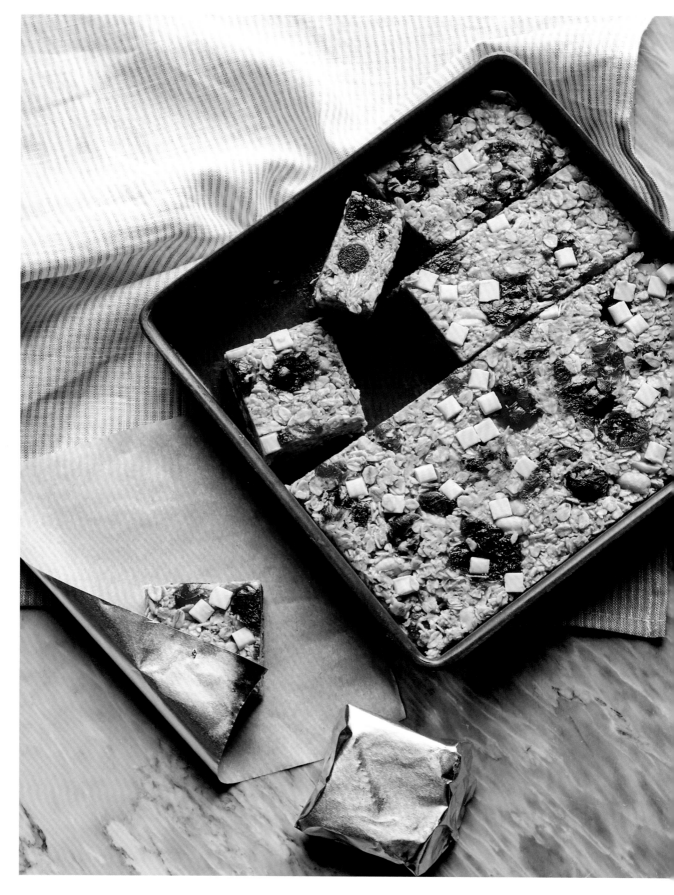

CHERRY, COCONUT AND WHITE CHOC ENERGY BARS

These are simple to make and so much nicer than shop-bought bars.

They freeze really well too, so can be made up and stored. They're also great as a dessert, chopped up and mixed with some fresh raspberries and yoghurt.

Makes 16

240 g (9 oz) gluten-free oats

60 g (2½ oz) toasted coconut plus
1 tablespoon for topping

1 teaspoon salt

200 g (7 oz) glace cherries, chopped

100 g (3½ oz) dried bitter cherries

100 g (3½ oz) peanuts

20 g (¾ oz) chia seeds

90 g (3½ oz) runny honey

80 g (3 oz) white chocolate

80 g (3 oz) coconut oil

120 g (4 oz) nut butter

1. Line a 20 x 20 cm (8 x 8 in) tray with greaseproof paper.

2. Mix all the dry ingredients together and set them aside.

3. Mix the honey, white chocolate, coconut oil and nut butter together, and warm gently until melted.

4. Either in a mixer or by hand, mix the dry and wet ingredients together.

5. Pour the mixture into the lined tray and press down firmly. Sprinkle the remaining coconut over the top.

6. Refrigerate for two hours then cut into squares. Store in the fridge for up to seven days.

Nutrition per serving:

Energy: 329 kcal | Total carbohydrate: 33 g (of which sugars: 18 g)

Fat: 18 g | Fibre: 5 g | Protein: 6.4 g | Salt: 0.46 g

GRAVELLY ROAD

Flavour fatigue is very prevalent amongst ultra-endurance riders, so let's keep it interesting with a bar in which every bite is different.

With the ever-growing popularity of gravel biking, it only seems right to name this version of rocky road after the sport and the inclusion of cocoa nibs does give it a distinctive gravelly feel.

Makes 16

200 g (7 oz) 70 per cent chocolate

100 g (3½ oz) 40 per cent chocolate

125 g (4 oz) unsalted butter

2 tablespoons golden syrup

1 tablespoon blackstrap molasses

100 g (3½ oz) Biscoff biscuits, crushed

80 g (3 oz) large marshmallows, cut into chunks

75 g (3 oz) glace morello cherries

75 g (3 oz) golden raisins

50 g (2 oz) cocoa nibs

pinch of sea salt flakes

1. Line a 20 x 20 cm (8 x 8 in) tray with greaseproof paper.
2. Melt the chocolate, butter, golden syrup and molasses together in a large bowl, over a pan of boiling water.
3. Stir in the rest of the ingredients, reserving the coco nibs and salt.
4. Pour the mix into the tray and smooth over the top with a spatula.
5. Sprinkle on the coco nibs and sea salt.
6. Refrigerate until set and then cut into squares.

Nutrition per serving:
Energy: 269 kcal | Total carbohydrate: 27 g (of which sugars: 21 g)
Fat: 16 g | Fibre: 2.1 g | Protein: 2.7 g | Salt: 0.18 g

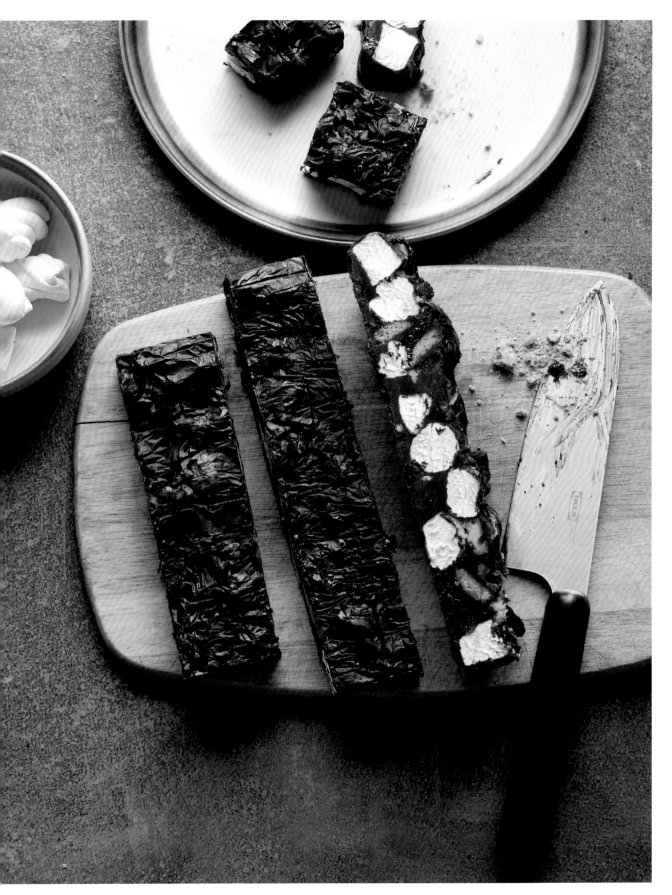

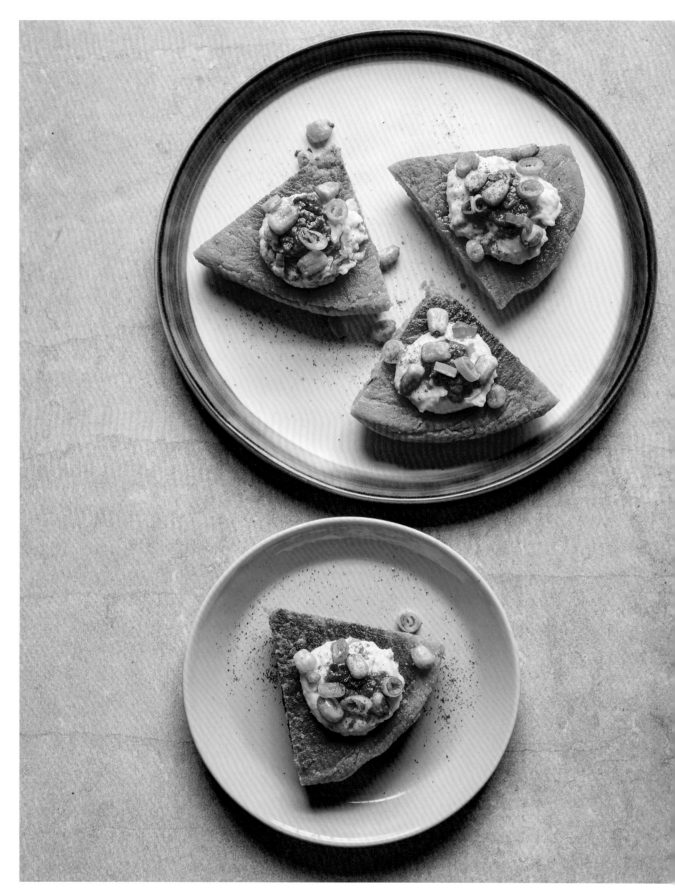

SWEET POTATO 'TATTIE SCONES'

Here's a modern twist on a Scottish breakfast favourite, the tattie scone, but these potato-based flatbreads are brought bang up to date with the inclusion of the sweet potato.

This is a fabulously rich source of complex carbohydrates (and if you can source purple sweet potatoes then so much the better).

Makes 8

300 g (11 oz) mashed sweet potato

200 g (7 oz) mashed Desirée potato

50 g (2 oz) butter, melted

1 teaspoon smoked paprika

1 teaspoon harissa paste

1 teaspoon sea salt flakes

1 egg

1 teaspoon baking powder

125 g (4 oz) plain flour

150 g (5 oz) grated sweet potato

1 teaspoon smoked garlic, chopped

4 tablespoons olive oil

Nutrition per serving:
Energy: 253 kcal | Total carbohydrate: 27 g (of which sugars: 5.8 g)
Fat: 14 g | Fibre: 2.4 g | Protein: 3.8 g | Salt: 0.71 g

1. Combine the mashed sweet potato and potato – total cooked weight 500 g (1 lb 2 oz) – with the butter, paprika, harissa, salt and egg.

2. Mix the baking powder and flour together, and incorporate them into the mash mix.

3. Lightly cook the grated sweet potato and smoked garlic in the olive oil.

4. Mix the grated sweet potato into the mash mix.

5. In true 'granny style', roll the dough into a large disc and use a 22 cm (9 in) plate or bowl to cut out a large disc approximately 5 mm ($\frac{1}{4}$ in) thick. Cut into four triangles – the shape is traditional for a tattie scone – then re-roll the trim and cut into another four triangles.

6. To cook, lightly grease a large frying pan and pan-fry each scone for 2–3 minutes on each side, turning once, to get them golden brown. Alternatively, if you want them to be firmer you can bake them in the oven for a little longer.

7. These can be served with sweet or savoury toppings – try jam or hummus, although not on the same scone unless you're a culinary savage.

CHOCOLATE CHERRY PANCAKE ROLLS

These cherry pancakes are not too sweet and can be a nice change as an on-the-bike snack or the base for a hearty breakfast.

Ideally, make up the batter the night before you want to use it. The recipe makes plenty and it will last for up to four days in the fridge. Alternatively, batch-cook the pancakes and freeze them for later.

Makes 6

4 eggs

250 ml (1 cup) chocolate milk

190 g (6¾ oz) gluten-free self-raising flour

40 g (1½ oz) bitter cocoa powder

35 g (1¼ oz) dried bitter cherries, finely chopped

50 g (2 oz) cocoa nibs

6 dessert spoons good-quality cherry jam

olive oil for frying

For breakfast

180 g (6 oz) frozen morello cherries

1 tablespoon brown sugar

1 teaspoon vanilla extract

6 tablespoons full fat Greek yoghurt

Nutrition per serving (pancake):
Energy: 346 kcal | Total carbohydrate: 40 g (of which sugars: 14 g)
Fat: 14 g | Fibre: 3.8 g | Protein: 12 g | Salt: 0.49 g

Nutrition per serving (pancake and toppings):
Energy: 431 kcal | Total carbohydrate: 49 g (of which sugars: 23 g)
Fat: 17 g | Fibre: 4 g | Protein: 17 g | Salt: 0.57 g

1. Whisk the eggs and chocolate milk together.

2. Mix the flour and cocoa powder together.

3. Gradually incorporate the flour mix into the egg mix, ensuring there are no lumps, and stir in the chopped cherries and cocoa nibs.

4. Refrigerate for at least 60 minutes.

5. To cook, heat a little oil in a 25 cm (10 in) non-stick pan, ladle in the pancake mix – this recipe makes large pancakes – and turn after 60 seconds.

6. Make sure you stir the pancake mix each time you cook a pancake to ensure even distribution of the cherries and cocoa nibs.

7. To make up for riding, spread the cherry jam evenly over the pancakes, roll up and wrap.

8. If a breakfast vibe is your thing, mix the frozen cherries, sugar and vanilla, and cook over a medium heat until the cherries have broken down and the juices have reduced. Serve up the pancakes with a good splodge of the cherry sauce and a spoonful of yoghurt.

TORTILLA WRAP TOASTIES

Once you discover the wrap as a toastie you will never look back.

Simple and delicious, they're just fabulous with some homemade Frei-speed falafels (see page 106) or hummus and some strong cheddar cheese. Just make sure you get the fold right if you're taking them on your ride.

Makes 2

2 large tortilla wraps

150 g (5 oz) falafels

1 tablespoon hummus

40 g ($1\frac{1}{2}$ oz) cheddar cheese, grated

2 teaspoons sweet chilli sauce

Nutrition per serving:
Energy: 242 kcal | Total carbohydrate: 25 g (of which sugars: 3.3 g)
Fat: 11 g | Fibre: 3.7 g | Protein: 8.9 g | Salt: 0.89 g

1. Preheat your toasted sandwich-maker.
2. Lay out a wrap, squash the falafels and press them down in one quarter of it.
3. Add some hummus and grated cheese.
4. Fold in half and then in half again.
5. Place it in the toasted sandwich maker for 3–4 minutes and serve with the sweet chilli sauce.

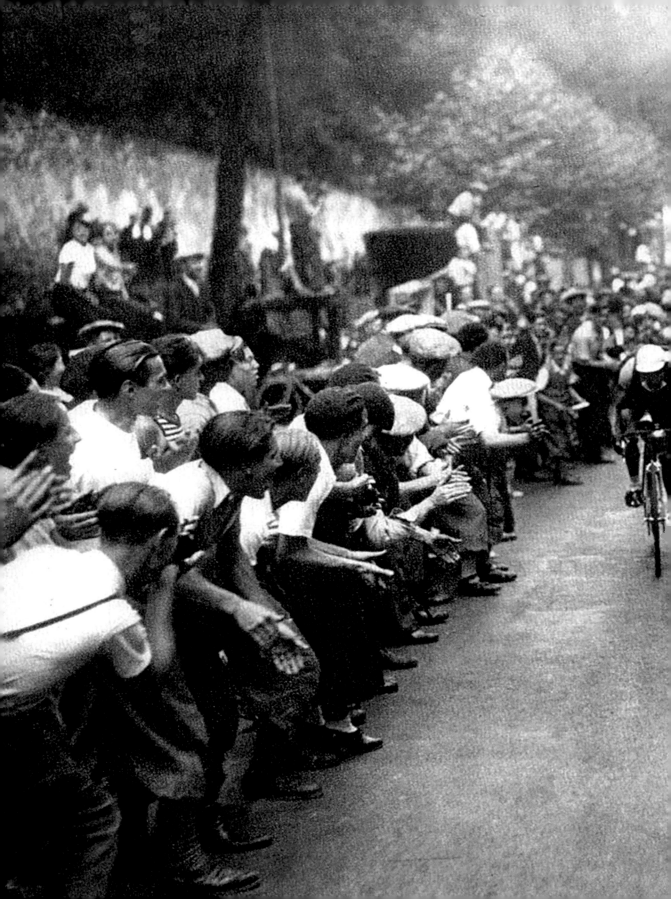

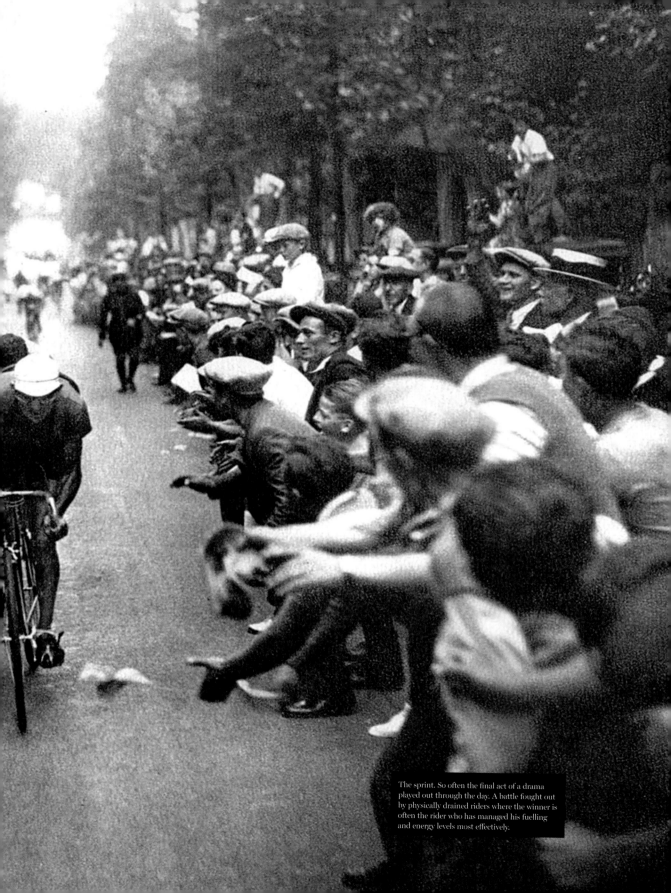

The sprint. So often the final act of a drama played out through the day. A battle fought out by physically drained riders where the winner is often the rider who has managed his fuelling and energy levels most effectively.

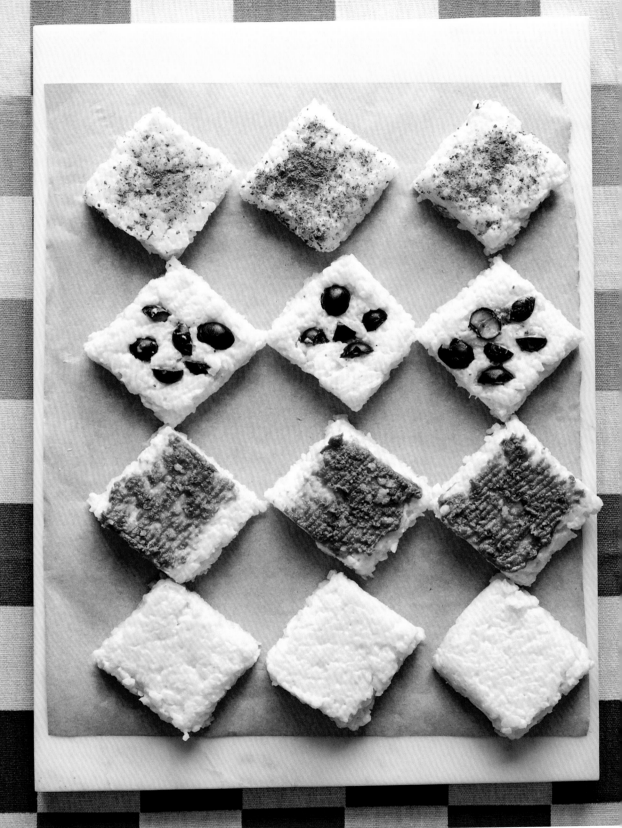

PRO RIDER RICE CAKES

Very much a staple ride food in the pro ranks, amateur cyclists rarely seem to use rice cakes, which is crazy, because they're easy to digest, rich in carbs and robust.

They're usually made in their hotel rooms by overworked soigneurs using a rice cooker, mini bar fridge and food storage bags, which means there's no need for special equipment, and the ingredients are cheap and widely available. Here is my go-to maple syrup and cinnamon base recipe, followed by a couple of recipes for my favourite flavourings.

Makes 12

250 g (9 oz) risotto rice

600 ml (2$\frac{1}{2}$ cups) water

30 g (1$\frac{1}{4}$ oz) coconut oil

$\frac{1}{2}$ teaspoon cinnamon

30 g (1$\frac{1}{4}$ oz) sugar

150 g (5 oz) full fat cream cheese

3 tablespoons maple syrup

Nutrition per serving:
Energy: 155 kcal | Total carbohydrate: 22 g | (of which sugars: 5.2 g)
Fat: 6.5 g | Fibre: 0.5 g | Protein: 2.4 g | Salt: 0.08 g

1. Line a 20 x 20 cm (8 x 8 in) cake tin with greaseproof paper (or for absolute authenticity use a large Ziploc bag).

2. Place the risotto rice, water, coconut oil, cinnamon and sugar in a saucepan and bring to a simmer.

3. Once simmering, cook over a low heat for 18 minutes until all the liquid has been absorbed.

4. While the mixture is still warm, stir in the cream cheese and maple syrup.

5. Spoon the mixture into the lined cake tin and press down evenly.

6. Refrigerate overnight (hotel mini bar fridge entirely optional) until set and then cut into squares.

HAM, PARMESAN AND FETA RICE CAKES

A savoury rice cake is an absolute must, because sweet flavour fatigue is a very real problem when on longer rides, training camps or stage races.

Fortunately, as well as all their other attributes, rice cakes are incredibly versatile.

Makes 12

250 g (9 oz) risotto rice

600 ml (2½ cups) water

30 g (1¼ oz) coconut oil

100 g (3½ oz) smoked ham, chopped

100 g (3½ oz) Parmesan, grated

75 g (3 oz) feta, crumbled

Nutrition per serving:
Energy: 156 kcal | Total carbohydrate: 16 g (of which sugars: 0 g)
Fat: 6.9 g | Fibre: 0.5 g | Protein: 7.1 g | Salt: 0.51 g

1. Line a 20 x 20 cm (8 x 8 in) cake tin with greaseproof paper.

2. Place the risotto rice, water and coconut oil in a saucepan and bring to a simmer.

3. Once simmering, cook over a low heat for 18 minutes until all the liquid has been absorbed.

4. While the mixture is still warm, stir in the smoked ham, Parmesan and feta.

5. Spoon the mixture into the lined cake tin and press down evenly.

6. Refrigerate overnight until set and then cut into squares.

SPECTACULAR SPECULOOS RICE CAKES

Speculoos are crunchy cookies that hail from the cycling heartland of Belgium.

In the UK and US, the speculoos spread is known as Biscoff spread and it's about the most addictive thing ever put in a jar. Rice cakes flavoured with this heaven-sent ingredient are pretty addictive, too.

Makes 12

250 g (9 oz) risotto rice

600 ml (2½ cups) water

30 g (1¼ oz) coconut oil

½ teaspoon cinnamon

150 g (5 oz) full fat cream cheese

225 g (8 oz) Biscoff spread

Nutrition per serving:
Energy: 229 kcal | Total carbohydrate: 32 g (of which sugars: 12 g)
Fat: 11 g | Fibre: 0.5 g | Protein: 2 g | Salt: 0.08 g

1. Line a 20 x 20 cm (8 x 8 in) cake tin with greaseproof paper.

2. Place the risotto rice, water, coconut oil and cinnamon in a saucepan and bring to a simmer.

3. Once simmering, cook over a low heat for 18 minutes until all the liquid has been absorbed.

4. While the mixture is still warm, stir in the cream cheese and Biscoff spread.

5. Spoon the mixture into the lined cake tin and press down evenly.

6. Refrigerate overnight until set and then cut into squares.

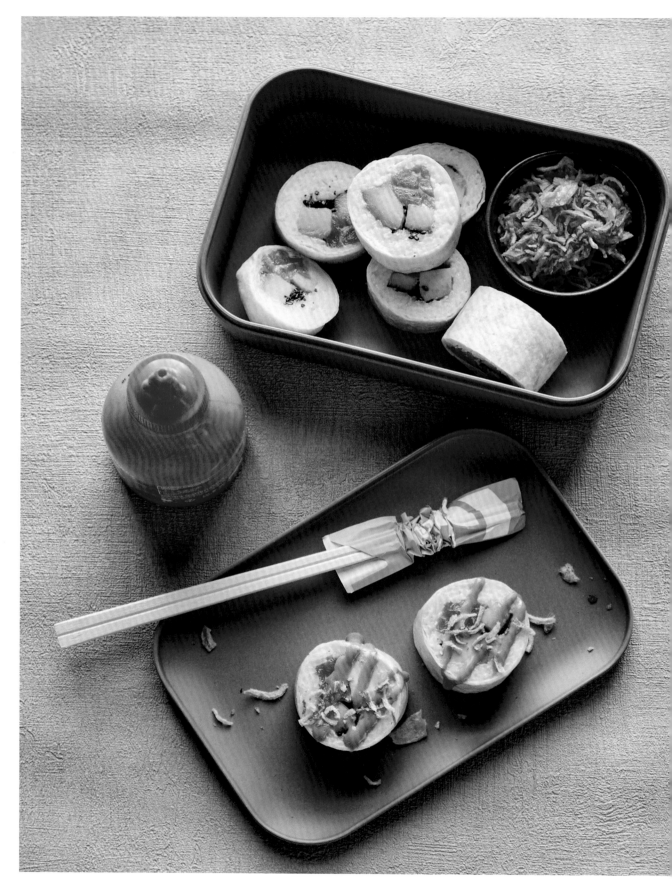

TORTILLA-WRAPPED SUSHI ROLLS

More carbs and more robust – just like the sushi you love, but using a tortilla wrap.

Does anyone really like soggy seaweed anyway? I always thought there must a better option to wrapping rice. Boom! Ride-resilient tortilla-wrapped sushi rolls. Sometimes I even surprise myself!

Makes 4

110 g ($3\frac{1}{2}$ oz) sushi rice

150 ml ($\frac{2}{3}$ cup) water

40 g ($1\frac{1}{2}$ oz) rice vinegar

35 g ($1\frac{1}{4}$ oz) white sugar

pinch of salt

2 large tortilla wraps

200 g (7 oz) fresh salmon, cut into long thin strips

$\frac{1}{2}$ avocado, sliced, brushed with lemon juice to stop discolouration

$\frac{1}{2}$ cucumber, seeds removed, cut into long batons

pickled ginger

wasabi paste

Nutrition per serving (half wrap):
Energy: 388 kcal | Total carbohydrate: 48 g (of which sugars: 11 g)
Fat: 14 g | Fibre: 2.7 g | Protein: 16 g | Salt: 0.83 g

1. Wash the rice in cold running water.

2. Cook the rice in a rice cooker or place the rice and water in a pan, bring to the boil and simmer with the lid on for 10 minutes.

3. Remove from the heat and allow to sit for 20 minutes.

4. While this is a happening, warm the vinegar and sugar until the sugar dissolves.

5. When the rice is ready, spread it out evenly on a tray and then add the vinegar and sugar mix, folding through gently. Season with salt.

6. Cover and allow to cool, but don't refrigerate.

7. Lay out the tortilla wrap and spread the sushi rice evenly across the middle, (or 12 cm/$1\frac{1}{2}$ in) approximately from top to bottom.

8. In the middle of the rice, place a line of salmon, then avocado and then cucumber. Top with some pickled ginger.

9. Using your finger, smear a little wasabi along the bottom of the line of fish and veggies (but don't lick your finger afterwards).

10. Roll up sushi-style, then wrap in cling film to firm up. Store in the freezer for 15 minutes.

11. Remove from the freezer and cut in half if you want a caveman portion or, alternatively, into large, bite-size chunks. Eat on the day you make it.

TERIYAKI TEMPEH

Tempeh is tofu's cousin – the same but different.

It's higher in protein, fermented, so it's good for gut health, and more similar in texture to meat if you're looking for a substitute. Boxed up, this makes a substantial on-the-road refueller, although it's also proper delicious in a wrap.

Makes 4

50 g (2 oz) teriyaki sauce

200 g (7 oz) tempeh

1 teaspoon olive oil

80 g (3 oz) cooked sushi race (see recipe for tortilla-wrapped sushi rolls, page 56)

1 tablespoon fresh coriander

Nutrition per serving:
Energy: 237 kcal | Total carbohydrate: 27 g (of which sugars: 3.5 g)
Fat: 6.5 g | Fibre: 5.8 g | Protein: 15 g | Salt: 2 g

1. Cut the tempeh into chunks. Place in a non-stick pan and fry in the oil until golden brown.

2. Add the teriyaki sauce and cook until well glazed.

3. Serve with the sushi rice and sprinkle over the coriander.

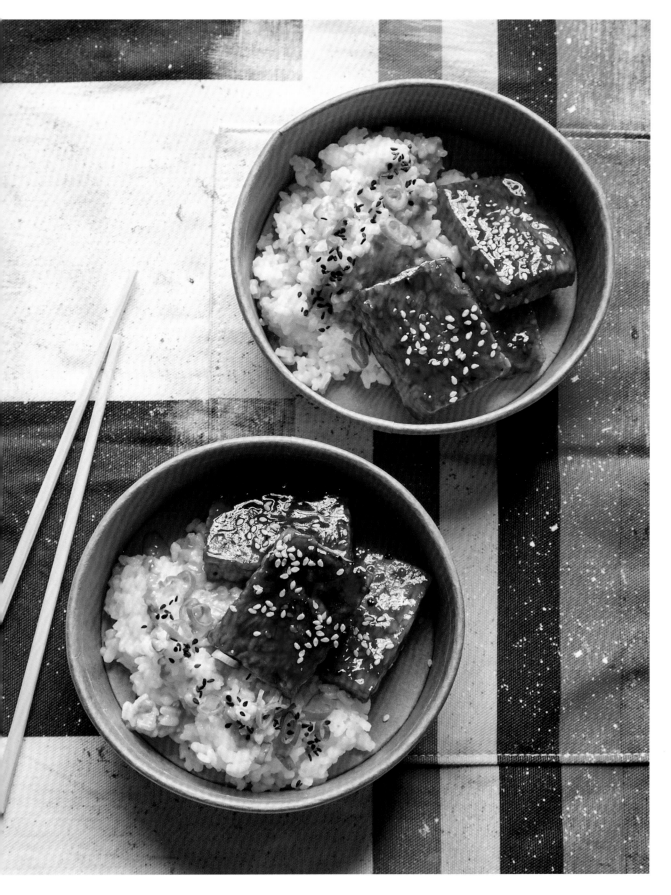

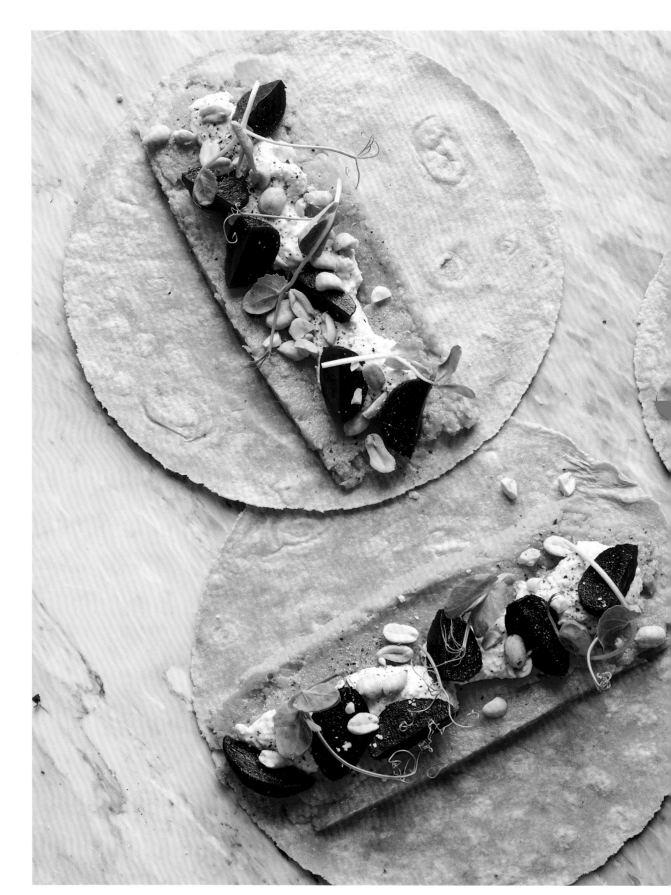

SWEET POTATO WRAPS WITH PEANUT HUMMUS AND ROASTED BEETS

How much goodness can you throw into one wrap?

Plenty of sweetness, some salt, some creaminess, some crunch – the flavours and textures going on here are mega! Here some of the big stars of the slow-release carb world come together in a wrap that will keep you rolling for hours.

Makes 2

2 large wraps or ideally sweet potato wraps

90 g ($3\frac{1}{2}$ oz) cooked sweet potato, crushed

2 tablespoons hummus

1 tablespoon salted peanuts

30 g ($1\frac{1}{4}$ oz) cooked beets, diced

A few stems of watercress as pictured (optional)

1. Spread the sweet potato on the wraps.

2. Add a layer of hummus and sprinkle on the peanuts.

3. Then throw on the beets in a cheffy fashion. Rock 'n' roll!

Nutrition per serving:

Energy: 279 kcal | Total carbohydrate: 25 g (of which sugars: 8.5 g)

Fat: 14 g | Fibre: 9.5 g | Protein: 7.8 g | Salt: 0.85 g

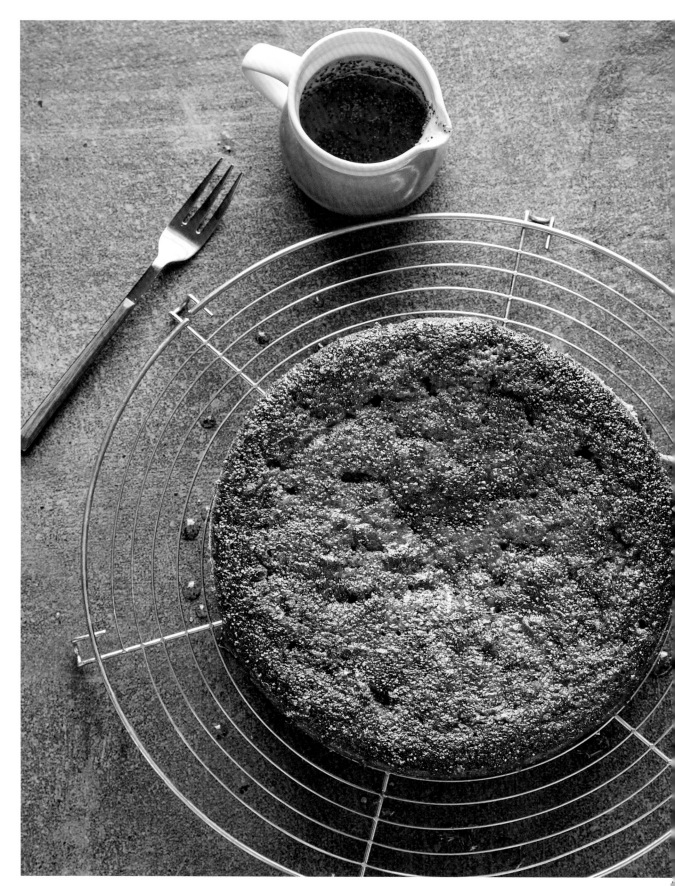

POLENTA AND POPPYSEED CAKE

When you're getting bored with your back-pocket provisions, try one of these zesty, seedy delights.

The gluten-free polenta gives them a soft texture that aids digestion when the going gets tough.

Makes 12

300 g (11 oz) soft unsalted butter

300 g (11 oz) golden Demerara sugar

juice and zest of 1 lime

juice and zest of 1 orange

4 eggs

300 g (11 oz) ground almonds

seeds from 2 cardamom pods, crushed

2 tablespoons poppyseeds

150 g (5 oz) polenta

1 teaspoon baking powder

Glaze

juice and zest of 1 orange

75 g (3 oz) brown sugar

icing sugar for dusting

Nutrition per serving:
Energy: 556 kcal | Total carbohydrate: 45 g (of which sugars: 34 g)
Fat: 37 g | Fibre: 2.4 g | Protein: 11 g | Salt: 0.19 g

1. Preheat your oven to 160°C/325°F/Gas 3, and line and grease a 20 x 20 cm (8 x 8 in) baking tray or cake tin.

2. Place the butter, sugar, and lime and orange zests into the bowl of a mixer and use the whisk attachment to beat until light and creamy.

3. Add the eggs, ground almonds, cardamom, poppy seeds, polenta, lime and orange juice, and baking powder, and beat again.

4. Pour the mixture into the lined baking tray and bake for 50–60 minutes. Allow to cool while making the glaze.

5. To make the glaze, put the orange juice, zest and sugar into a pan and simmer until it becomes a light syrup. When the cake is cool, prick the top with a fork and spoon over the glaze.

6. To serve, dust with icing sugar or sprinkle a teaspoon of poppy seeds over the top.

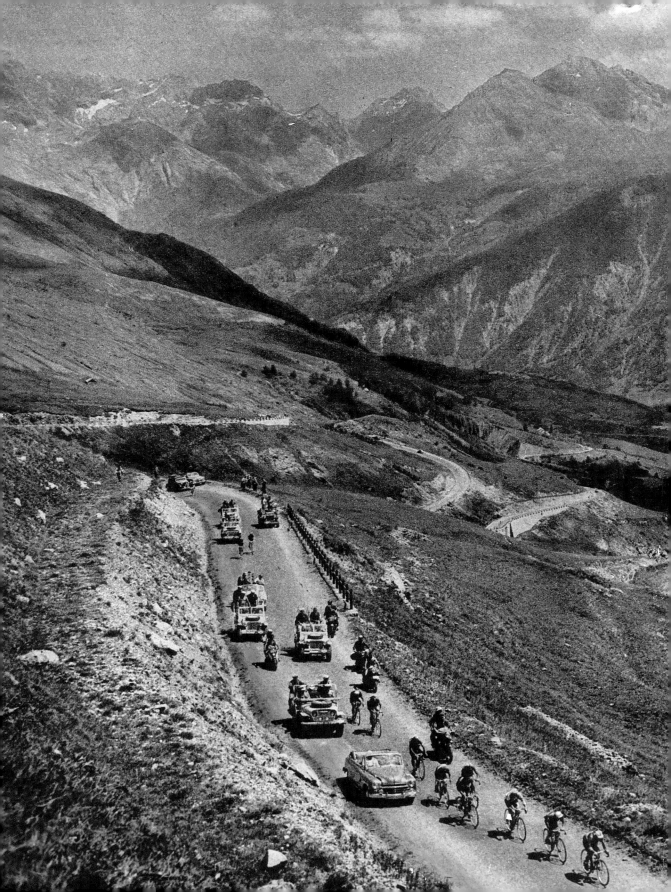

PORTABLES PRACTICALITIES

If you're the kind of cyclist who likes your Rapha jersey to hang smooth you're not going to like this, because nearly everything has to go in your pockets. Unsightly bulges and bumps provide a good guessing game for anyone following your wheel, but that's the price you pay for packing real and tasty food on your ride. On the plus side, though, it's amazing just how much you can fit in those pockets!

Riding in the mountains presents unique nutritional challenges. The arduous and frequent climbs require a pre-race, on-the-bike and post-race plan for sustenance and hydration.

Before you pack, make an inventory of what you need. How many rice cakes, snacks, bars or gels will you be carrying? A mental list will stop you rooting around for that last gel when you had it an hour ago.

There are a few practical issues concerning food in your pockets. First, particularly when you have your eyes on the road and a grip on the handlebars, it needs to be easily accessible. If you know where your food and gels are stored you won't have to forage around desperately. Most important is stability on the bike. If you're right-handed, then keep that hand on your handlebars. Use your left to reach back and grab. Obviously, if you are left-handed, then the opposite is true. If you're reaching back with your left hand, then the easiest pocket to reach is the left hip pocket. This is where your food needs to be stashed. Use the middle pocket for your rain jacket, arm warmers or gilet and a mini-pump if it isn't fixed. The right pocket can house anything you might need when you stop: credit card, keys or maybe a phone.

Before you pack, make an inventory of what you need. How many rice cakes, snacks, bars or gels will you be carrying? A mental list will stop you rooting around for that last gel when you had it an hour ago. Make sure anything sticky, moist or delicate is wrapped well. The last thing you need is a handful of mush, a pocketful of crumbs or a muffin covered in fluff. And remember, it is going to get hot and sweaty back there. Ensure the food will not fall out, but is also easy to open with one hand. Check out YouTube for some good advice on wrapping rice cakes or similar items. It's just a few folds of foil, but worth having a technique if it keeps things fresh. If you're taking bars you've bought, you might also want to snip the tops off the wrappers to make them easier to open as you pedal. Go careful doing this with gels, though, as they could leak and leave a real mess.

Of course, readymade products are convenient and serve their purpose, but it's just more crap to go to landfill. One of the advantages of making your own food or gels is that you can use environmentally friendly or recyclable packaging. There are a few different ways you can do this. I like to use foil-backed greaseproof paper, which I keep to reuse next time, but beeswax wraps and bags are also ideal. Hygienic and easy to clean, if they look like they're wearing out and don't seal, just pop them in an oven at the lowest temperature for a couple of minutes and hold them until they dry. Even better, take inspiration from Olympic silver medallist mountain biker Sina Frei. During the off-season she sews her own colourful little snack bags to take on the bike or give to her friends.

IN THE BAG

If you've got a small under-saddle bag there might be room to wedge in a bar next to your spare inner tube and tyre levers, but bear in mind you'll need to stop to retrieve it, so it might be wise to save the space for the real emergency rations. More useful is a bag, often called a bar bag, that you attach to your handlebars, or a box, often called a bento box, that you attach to your top tube. These fix on either with Velcro straps or Braze-on bolts if you have them.

Bento boxes are only really necessary for a long ride, but can be really useful. They are very popular with triathletes, and ultra-endurance cyclists and gravel riders seem to have taken to them, too. They come in various sizes, keep food dry and fresh rather than allowing it to get sweaty or crushed, and they can save you from having a scone wedged against your back for a hundred kilometres. Don't worry about aerodynamics. They have a very streamlined shape and if you position them correctly (preferably snug against the stem) they contribute a negligible drag. They are also easily accessed, with large zip-pulls that you can manipulate even wearing gloves, or magnetic flip-top lids which open and shut without any fuss.

One other investment you might consider is a gel flask. These are especially useful if you make your own energy gels. A small one can hold the equivalent of five sachets and saves you the hassle of opening a gel on the road or having to put a half-consumed, leaking sachet back into your pocket. They will fit neatly into the back of your jersey and come in an easily squeezable soft shell.

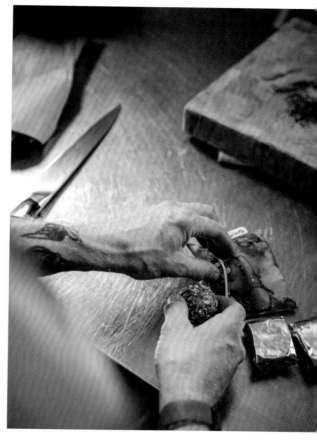

Little balls of sweet or savoury goodness are just perfect for your snack bag.

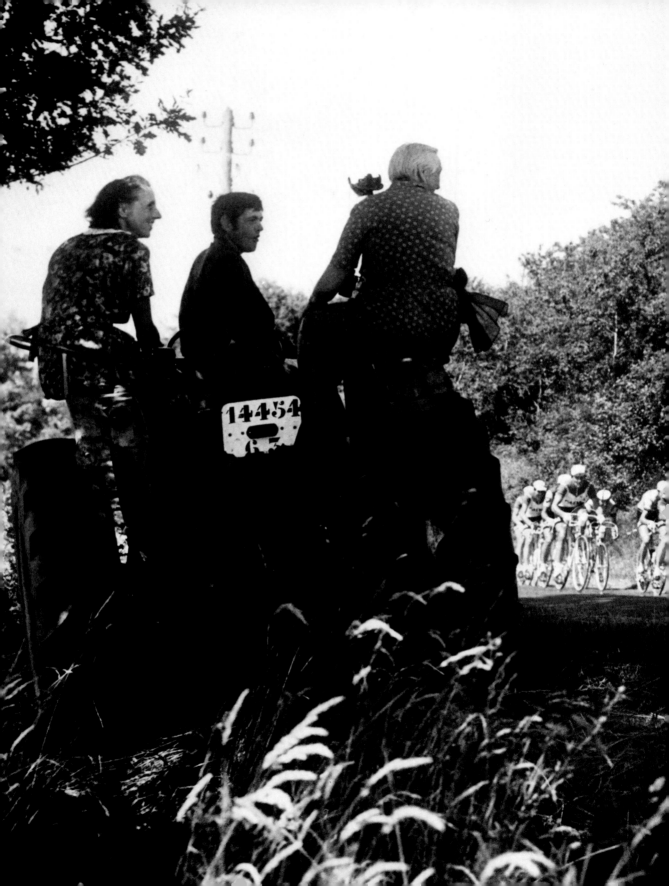

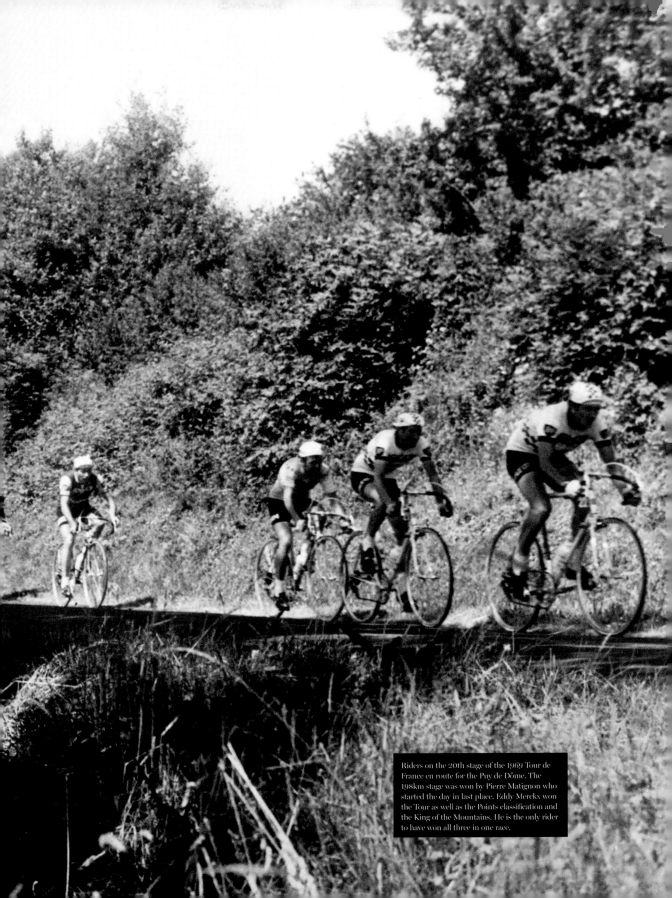

Riders on the 20th stage of the 1969 Tour de France en route for the Puy de Dôme. The 198km stage was won by Pierre Matignon who started the day in last place. Eddy Merckx won the Tour as well as the Points classification and the King of the Mountains. He is the only rider to have won all three in one race.

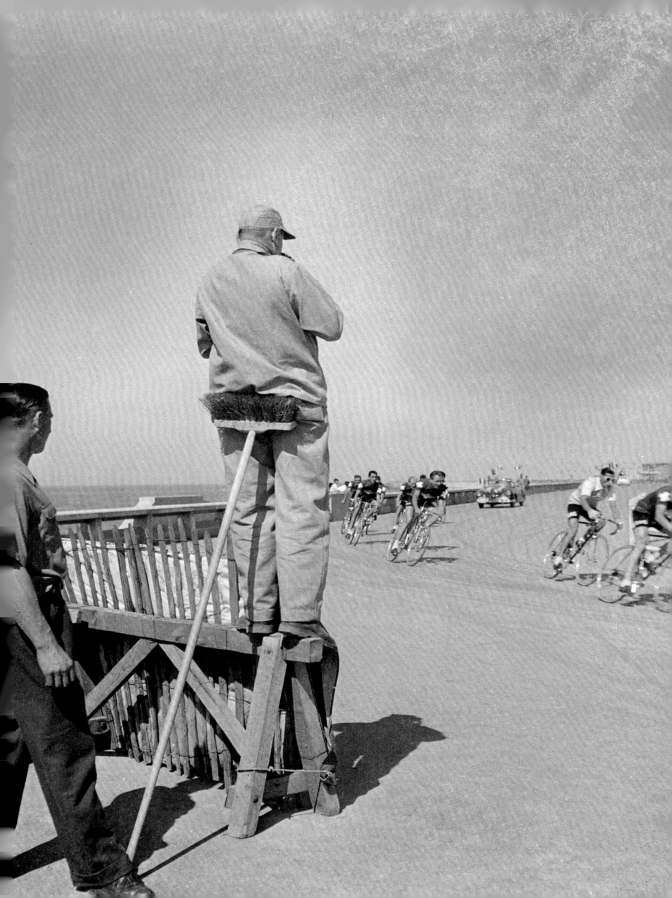

STROOPWAFELS

It's Belgian for energy waffle. Well, OK, stroopwafel translates as 'syrup waffle', but it could be. Cyclists in the Low Countries have reached for them to give them back their oomph for years, and now the secret is well and truly out. It could be the instant hit from the glucose in the syrup or the slower acting complex carbs of the biscuit – or perhaps the 'back pocket oven' warms the caramel to just the right level of gooeyness. Either way, it can give you a waffly big boost just when you need it.

The café stop has been part of cycling culture forever. A chance to get off the saddle and chill. A coffee, an unhurried opportunity to answer the call of nature and maybe even a cake to set you on your way…

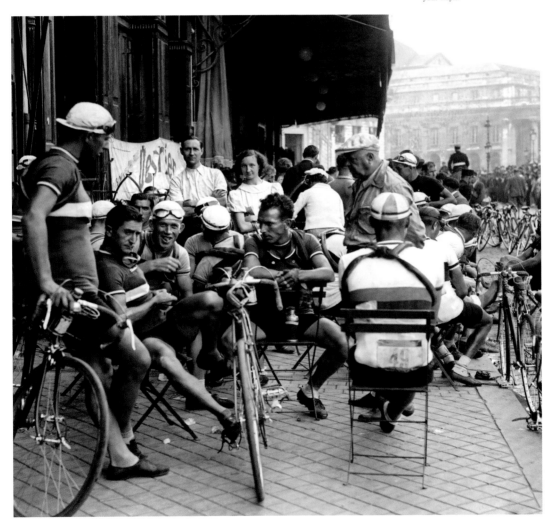

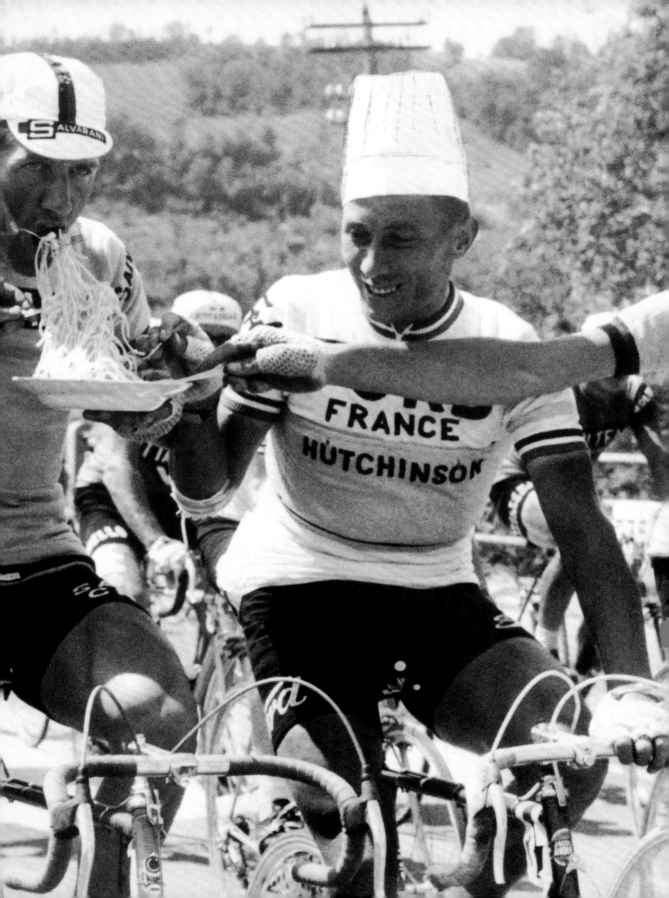

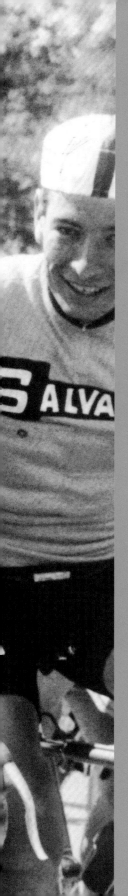

RECIPES
CARBS ARE KING

There's no point setting off with an empty tank. Carbs are what cyclists run on – as I've said before, they're our fuel – and whether you're filling up at breakfast (my English breakfast muffin toast – see page 86 – will give you an ideal start to the day) or dinner (Ghetto paella – see page 82 – should hit the spot), these recipes will help you power on when the road ahead is long and grippy.

Vittorio Adorni, Jacques Anquetil and Felice Gimondi taking feeding on-the-bike all too literally during the Giro D'Italia in 1966. From carbo-loading to energy gels to nutritional periodisation, fuelling has developed rapidly since those days.

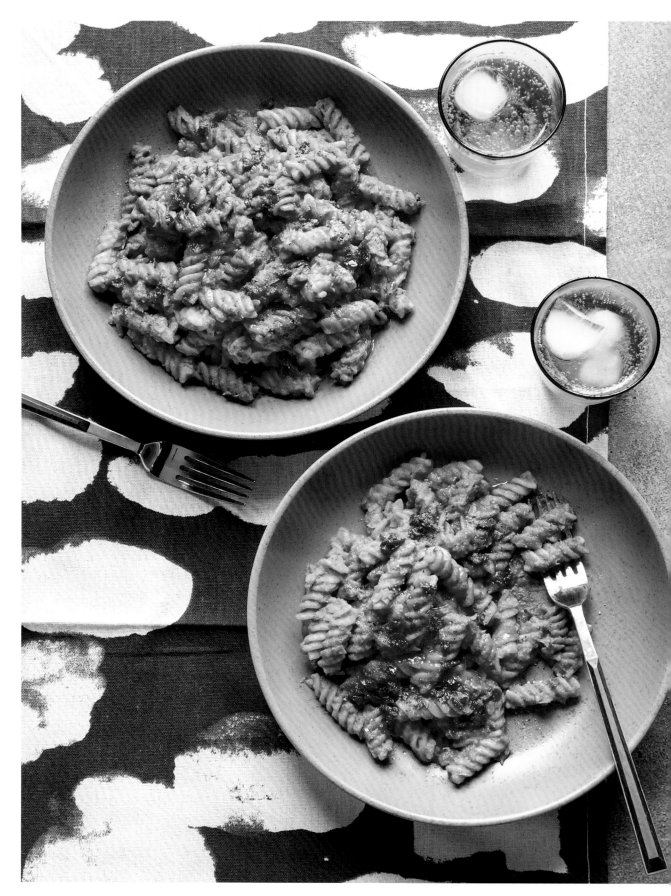

DEATH WISH PASTA

This pasta with sauce is proper food, but it contains no dairy, meat or fish, so it won't go off, even if it's hanging around all day in your bar bag.

Make it up the night before an epic ride and enjoy a decent protein hit and some savoury carby goodness.

Serves 2

200 g (7 oz) fusilli pasta

246g (9 oz) cooked butter beans

100 g (3½ oz) sun dried tomatoes

2 tablespoons tomato purée

2 teaspoons harissa paste

2 teaspoons red miso paste

1 teaspoon smoked paprika

1 teaspoon turmeric

1 teaspoon sea salt flakes

2 tablespoons extra virgin olive oil

125 ml (½ cup) pasta water

Nutrition per serving:
Energy: 884 kcal | Total carbohydrate: 89 g (of which sugars: 8.7 g)
Fat: 44 g | Fibre: 18 g | Protein: 22 g | Salt: 4 g

1. Add the pasta to a pan of boiling salted water to cook.

2. In a blender, add all the ingredients apart from the pasta water and blend to make a smooth paste.

3. When the pasta is cooked, and before straining it, add the measured starchy pasta water to the purée.

4. Strain the pasta, return to the pan, add the purée and adjust the seasoning if necessary. This can be eaten straightaway or cooled and refrigerated ahead of a big day's riding.

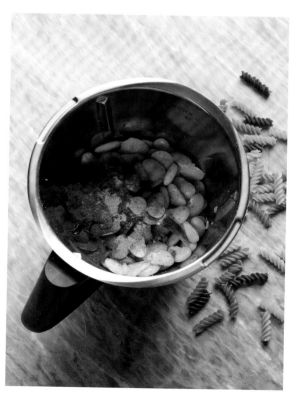

SWEET POTATO WAFFLES

Despite the name, this is a savoury waffle, but it's just as good as the sweet version.

In fact, the carbtastic sweet potato works a treat in these snacks, but the regular spud will do just as well – it's your call. If you don't have a waffle machine, these can be cooked in a pan too.

Makes 4

330 g (11½ oz) mashed sweet potato

270 ml (1 cup) semi-skimmed milk

1 large egg

100 g (3½ oz) gluten-free flour

1 teaspoon bicarbonate of soda

salt and pepper

spray oil

Nutrition per serving:

Energy: 216 kcal | Total carbohydrate: 38 g (of which sugars: 13 g)

Fat: 3.1 g | Fibre: 2.7 g | Protein: 7.6 g | Salt: 0.22 g

1. Make sure the mashed potato is cool and whisk the milk into it.

2. Mix in the egg.

3. Mix the flour and bicarb together and whisk them into the potato mix. Season well.

4. Preheat your waffle-maker and spray the plates with oil. Cook the waffles then cool them on a cooling rack.

Make a meal of it

These are great with crushed avocado and smoked salmon on top.

BANGING GULAB JAMUN

The famous Indian festival dessert – a fried sweet dumpling – is the inspiration for this delicious doughnut-style energy booster.

However, thanks to the air fryer, there's no dripping oil here, and I've snuck in some protein powder too. It's just about as far removed from a commercial doughnut as you can get.

Makes 12

Base dough

125 g (4 oz) gluten-free flour

30 g (1¼ oz) ground almonds

15 g (½ oz) desiccated coconut

1 teaspoon baking powder

½ teaspoon ground cardamom

½ teaspoon allspice

½ teaspoon turmeric

½ teaspoon ground cinnamon

70 g (3 oz) vanilla protein powder

75 g (3 oz) full fat Greek yoghurt

50 g (2 oz) butter, melted

3 tablespoons warm water

To finish

30 g (1¼ oz) caster sugar

1 teaspoon cinnamon

2 tablespoons good quality jam

Nutrition per serving:
Energy: 144 kcal | Total carbohydrate: 15 g (of which sugars 6.3g)
Fat: 6.4 g | Fibre: 0.7 g | Protein: 6.6 g | Salt: 0.24 g

1. Place all the dry ingredients into the bowl of a mixer and use the paddle attachment to mix them.

2. Mix in the Greek yoghurt and melted butter.

3. Gradually add the water until a nice dough forms.

4. Roll into 12 balls – each one should weigh around 35 g (1¼ oz) – spray with oil and cook in the air fryer at 170°C/340°F for 8 minutes.

5. Plunge the balls straight into the sugar and cinnamon, and when cool open them up get the jam in. Enjoy!

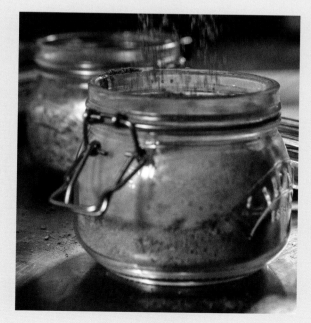

A handy selection of storage jars allows you to keep whatever you don't need for next time. Glass jars with clip tops are ideal, but Tupperware, steel and bamboo containers are all options. Best of all, clean and reuse your empty jam and peanut butter jars or spice bottles.

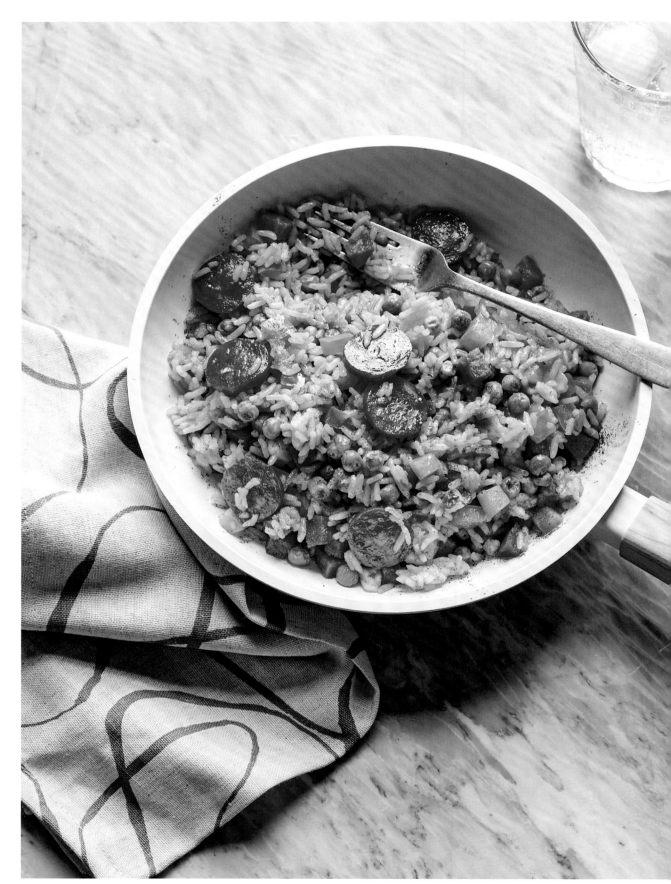

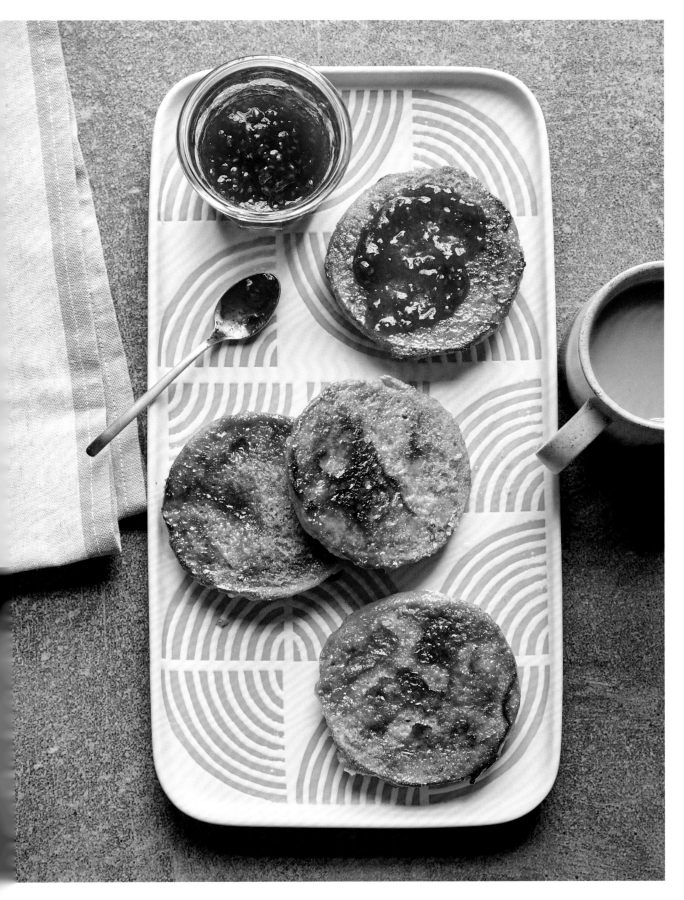

CIABATTA FIVE-MINUTE MINI PIZZAS

Using pre-made ciabatta is a no-fuss way to knock out the simplest of quick-fire pizzas with a topping of your choice.

We all know frozen is never the answer, but this solution to the pizza-in-a-hurry conundrum does tick all the boxes. Simple to prepare and ready to eat or chop it into bite-size pieces and take it with you.

Serves 3

One ciabatta loaf, approximately 300 g (11 oz)

1½ tablespoons olive oil

3 teaspoons basil pesto

3 tablespoons passata

120 g (4 oz) mozzarella, sliced

Optional toppings: anything you please (apart from pineapple – stay classy!)

Nutrition per serving:
Energy: 548 kcal | Total carbohydrate: 50 g (of which sugars: 5.2 g)
Fat: 29 g | Fibre: 4 g | Protein: 20 g | Salt: 1.8 g

1. Preheat the oven to 210°C/410°F/Gas 6.

2. Cut the loaf into 3 cm (1 in) slices. Brush one side with olive oil and place this side down on a non-stick tray.

3. Spread one teaspoon of basil pesto on each slice.

4. Then spread one tablespoon of passata on each slice.

5. Top each one with mozzarella.

6. Bake for 5–6 minutes until the cheese is melted and the base is nice and crispy. These are great as pre-made bike snacks, because the bread eats really well at room temperature.

HB SAUCE

This sauce is a favourite of US MTB rider Haley Batten and it makes a great base for an awesome salad.

Just mix it with pretty much any raw veg or stir it into cooked noodles or rice. Add some cooked garbanzo beans for a perfect ride food option or try it post-ride with Miso sesame salmon (see page 120) or Chicken Murch-nuggets (see page 110).

Serves 4

75 g (3 oz) peanut butter

1 tablespoon white wine vinegar

60 g (2½ oz) sweet chilli sauce

1 tablespoon soy sauce

1 tablespoon ketjap manis (Indonesian sweet soy sauce)

1 tablespoon extra virgin olive oil

Nutrition per serving:

Energy: 194 kcal | Total carbohydrate: 13 g (of which sugars: 11 g)
Fat: 13 g | Fibre: 1.3 g | Protein: 5.6 g | Salt: 1 g

1. Whisk all the ingredients together.

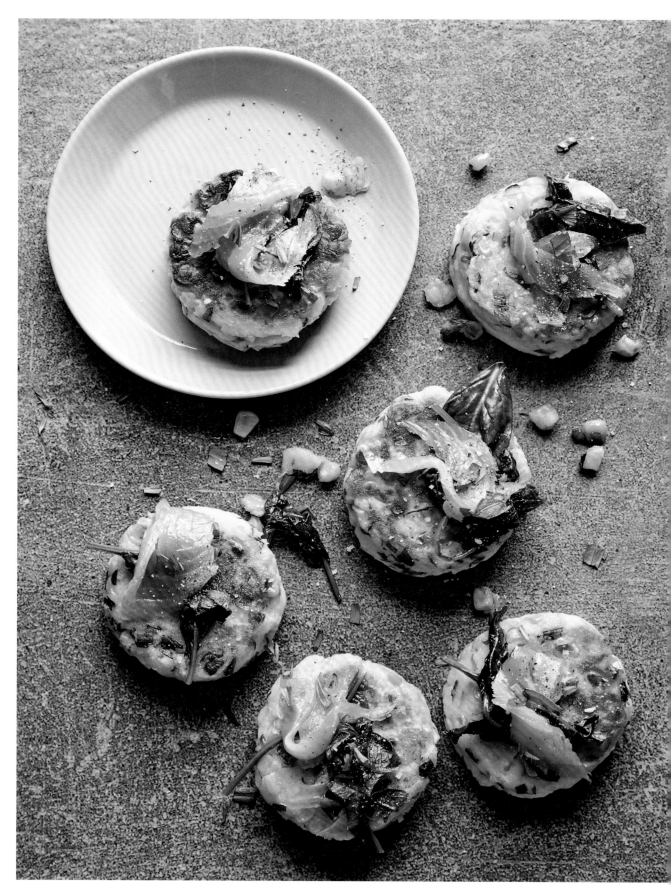

CARBY CORN CAKES

These corn cakes are perfect on-the-road fare – if you can resist eating them straight out of the pan, that is.

Just a few simple ingredients can be turned into a tasty and flexible base for many light meals. However, if you're making these for the bike, it's best to make them no bigger than 5 cm (2 in) across.

Makes 6

340 g (12 oz) sweetcorn

200 g (7 oz) dry mashed potato

100 g ($3\frac{1}{2}$ oz) gluten-free flour

1 medium egg

1 small bunch of chives/tarragon, chopped

salt and pepper

1 tablespoon olive oil

50 g (2 oz) unsalted butter

Nutrition per serving:
Energy: 228 kcal | Total carbohydrate: 26 g (of which sugars: 4.5 g)
Fat: 11 g | Fibre: 3 g | Protein: 4.9 g | Salt: 0.04 g

1. Preheat the oven to 190°C/375°F/Gas 5.

2. Mix the sweetcorn, potato, flour, egg and herbs together. Season well.

3. Mould into 7.5 cm (3 in) rounds, tidying them up using a pastry cutter.

4. Melt the oil and butter in a non-stick pan and colour both sides of the cakes.

5. Place them on a non-stick tray and bake for 8–10 minutes. They can be pre-cooked and stored in the fridge for three days.

Make a meal of it

Add grilled bacon or poached eggs and sautéed spinach. Would also work really well with smoked salmon and a squeeze of fresh lemon.

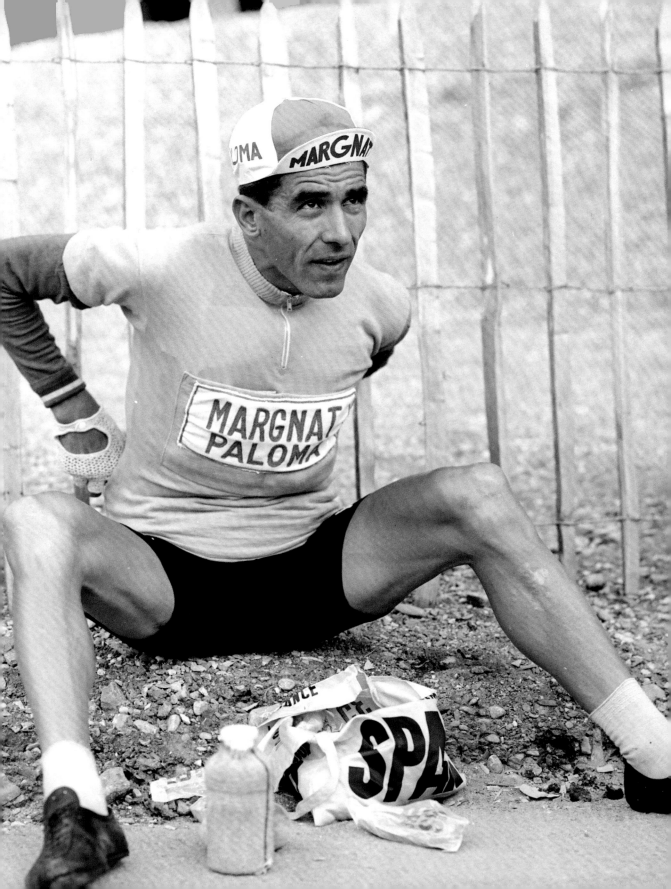

egg, mackerel and rice... the permutations are pretty endless.

Pantry dishes can be a godsend if you have a busy schedule, but fresh food – meat, fish, vegetables, fruit and dairy products – are key to any high-performance diet. We might be talking about an extra 15 minutes of preparation and a little longer cooking time, but that time will be well worth it when you're enjoying real food that helps you reach your nutrition and weight targets. Even then, I have plenty of tips that will help you minimise your time in the kitchen. Here are a few that are worth considering.

Don't peel Most vegetables and plenty of fruits (including kiwi fruit, which has fibre and nutrients galore) don't need peeling, and eating the skin delivers added nutritional value.

Chop, chop! Keep your knives sharp and chop vegetables, chicken and fish small to help them cook faster. Pre-chopped hard vegetables, such as carrots, peppers, broccoli and cauliflower florets, should be OK if you leave them in a container in the fridge for up to a week, while softer vegetables, such as tomatoes and cucumbers, can last three or four days.

Double up Make twice as much as you need and store it in the fridge or freezer for another meal. A bowlful of salad can make lunches or bolster up meals for a good half of the week, and a saucepan full of hearty homemade soup can be refrigerated or frozen for a meal in minutes.

Think ahead If you have time now, but not later, use that time wisely. Pre-cooked hard-boiled eggs and grilled chicken can both last a few days in the fridge.

Cook faster When time is of the essence, some techniques are quicker than others. Grilling, stir-frying and steaming are often quick and easy, and certainly better than waiting 20 minutes for the oven to heat up. The style of cooking has minimal effect on the nutritional content of the food, although as a general rule a shorter cooking time, a lower temperature and a smaller amount of water will give better nutritional results.

Plug in Nowhere will you find more time-saving devices than in the kitchen and you'd be a fool not to use them (if your electricity bill allows, of course). The smoothie-maker, toaster, rice cooker and air fryer can all help. A microwave is a lifesaver for its quick-cook baked potatoes, defrosting qualities and for warming up leftovers, while an old-fashioned pressure cooker is a great shortcut for cooking grains, legumes, stews and soups (nutritionally, the high temperature is cancelled out by the shorter cooking time).

While you were out So you get home starving after a day's ride, but are too exhausted to cook. No worries! Your meal is waiting for you. Another appliance that's worth considering purchasing (or getting out of the back of the cupboard) is a slow cooker, which can be one of the cyclist's best friends. A beef stew, vegan chilli or chicken tagine – all can be cooking away while you're out pushing the pedals. Come winter, a slow cooker can even turn your overnight oats into a warming breakfast.

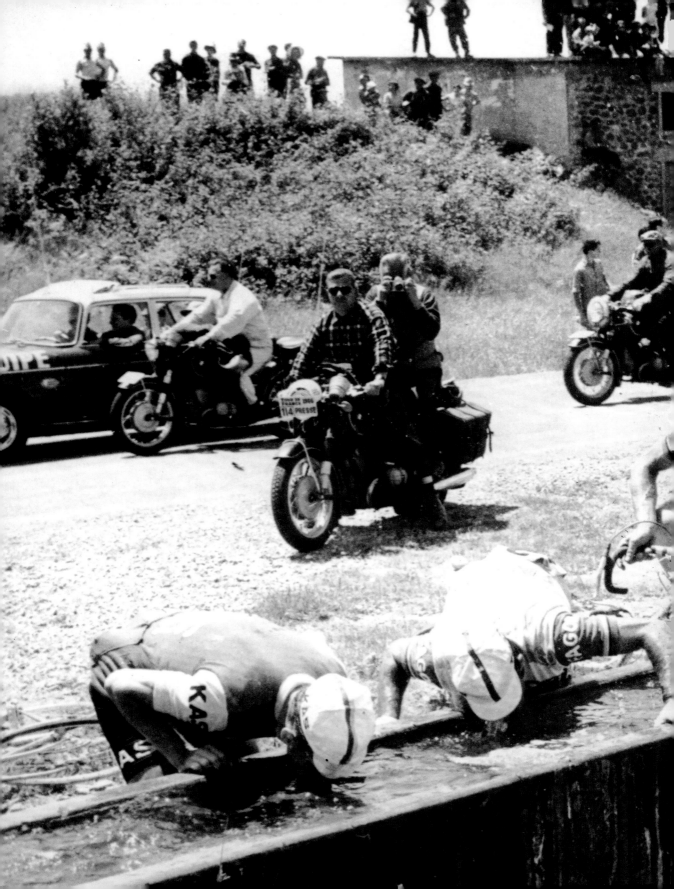

RECOVERY

How do you feel when you get back from a long, hard ride? Starving hungry and ready to eat the entire contents of the fridge along with the fridge itself? Is the thought of a short nap far more appealing than anything you've got in the larder? Or is your appetite traumatised by over-exertion and you can't even contemplate food let alone look at it? You've probably experienced all these scenarios at different times.

Rehydration 1950s style. Tour de France riders break to fill their bottles and drink straight from a long wooden trough during a sweltering stage of the 1958 race.

Before you dig into that mountain of food or glug that protein shake down in one, take a moment to calculate just how many calories you've expended, remembering to include the snacks and gels en route.

Cyclists are diverse folk and our refuelling requirements and desires are various, and can change from day to day. As we've seen elsewhere in this book, it's foolhardy to set any hard and fast rules, but guidelines, yep, we've got a few of those.

The first is just a polite wake-up call. Be honest. How hard a ride was that? Do you really need to refuel as if you'd been up both the Col de la Madeleine and the Télégraphe? Before you dig into that mountain of food or glug that protein shake down in one, take a moment to calculate just how many calories you've expended, remembering to include the snacks and gels en route. If you're not vigilant, you'll find the weight goes on easily, but it won't be so easy to shift.

THE THREE RS OF RECOVERY

Replenish Even if you have refuelled effectively during the ride, you may well have dug deep into your glycogen stores. The supplies in your liver and muscles will both need topping up and that means carbs. How much will depend on the level of your exertions and the proximity of your next hard ride.

Rehydrate It's a better than fair bet that after any reasonably prolonged exercise you will end up with a hydration deficit. You are unlikely – and probably unwise (see page 170) – to have drunk enough to replace all the fluid lost through sweat. Again, there is no need to down water like a man at a desert oasis. We don't just need fluid but salt and minerals to rehydrate safely and effectively.

Repair Our muscles have taken a right going-over during the day and they need some love and attention by way of protein. But they are not the only part of the body that needs nurturing, as the immune system needs bolstering with antioxidants.

THE ANABOLIC WINDOW

When cycling, your body is in a catabolic state where you are actively burning fuel to maintain energy levels – hence the need to refuel on the bike. Once you get off the bike, your body reverts to an anabolic state. This is the opposite, where the protein and carbs consumed are dedicated to building and repairing muscle tissue.

The anabolic window is a protein shake manufacturer's dream. What a marketing tool! The anabolic window supposedly means that there is a limited time – 45 minutes to an hour – after exercise when your body undergoes the repair and rebuild process, so when you've crossed the finish line chug that super-hydrolysed-complete-protein choco-fruity shake just as soon as you can!

Now to a certain extent this is true, but your system doesn't pull the shutters down at 45 minutes. Indeed, the window is now believed to be open for two or more hours, so there's no hurry, which means there's plenty of time to have a shower and consume some real food instead. Indeed, if you're not in a stage race and don't have a big ride the next day or another session a few hours later, there is much to be said for consuming nutrients over a period of several hours after exercise. The rate at which they are utilised may be slower, but the overall result will be the same.

BED AND BREAKFAST

On the other hand, the rate of protein synthesis – the speed at which your muscles repair themselves – is affected by several different factors, but one major one is fasting, notably when you are asleep. When the levels of available protein are low the body prioritises major organs like the liver and heart. This is why it helps to have slow digesting protein as your evening meal. This could include

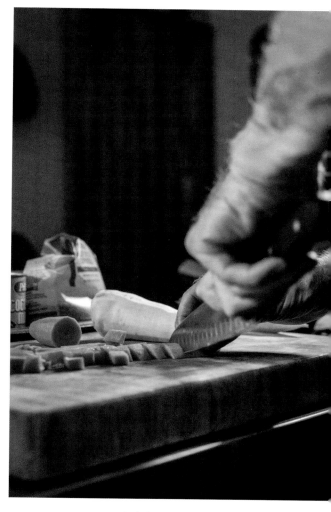

The rhythmic and focused chopping of vegetables can be a really calming and almost zen-like activity.

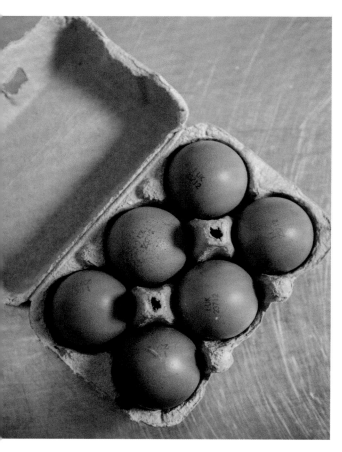

Eggs are surely the chef's best friend? Versatile, perfectly packaged, a protein booster and only one of two natural food sources that contain vitamin D.

eggs, poultry, fish, tofu, legumes and lentils, as well dairy products such as Greek yoghurt and cottage or ricotta cheese. Similarly, a protein-rich breakfast such as overnight oats, eggs, wheat cereal or a smoothie can help stimulate the process in the morning.

THE QUICK FIX

Let's face it, though, our lives are sometimes haphazard and chaotic. Often you might finish a ride and find yourself still hours from home, relying on what you left in the car or can pick up from a local store or café. Alternatively, you might arrive home looking for something that is quick and easy to prepare. The following, perhaps on toast or in a sandwich – two slices of wholemeal toast in themselves provide 40 g of carbohydrate, 8g of protein and a little fibre – can be on the table in minutes and will be enough to see you through that initial recovery period.

Eggs Scrambled, boiled or in an omelette, eggs are fantastically versatile and a great source of protein, as well as vitamins A and B and other nutrients. I always use free range.

Baked beans Cheap, quick and easy – no wonder beans on toast is many cyclists' go-to recovery snack. One small tin will give you around 25 g of carbs and 10 g of protein, which is well enough to set the recovery in motion.

Tinned fish Salmon, tuna, sardines or mackerel contain plenty of protein – around 25 g in a small tin – and they also contain omega 3, which can aid recovery by decreasing muscle inflammation.

Chicken Grilled or roasted chicken breast is a great option if you're looking for something unchallenging at the end of a tough ride. A few slices of thinly sliced chicken can provide around 20 g of protein.

Tofu Not just for vegetarian or vegan riders, tofu can offer a great protein-rich variation in a post-ride snack. It can be eaten raw, but is quickly grilled, baked or fried and is excellent with a little salad in a sandwich.

Cottage cheese The humble, lumpy, semi-solid cheese has emerged from the doldrums to take its rightful place in the pantheon of recovery sandwich fillings. You'll find 100 g provides just under 10 g of protein and it sits perfectly with fruit, salad or most of the above food items.

A FINAL NOTE ON RECOVERY DRINKS

The convenience and ease of refuelling with a ready-made drink is understandably attractive to many riders who are hot, dehydrated and exhausted at the end of a ride. A commercially produced drink is easily consumed and is theoretically designed to provide the carbs, protein and hydration required for rapid recovery. Many manufacturers play on the myth that you need to consume it more or less as soon as you're off the bike, but this is really your choice. There is nothing in these drinks that cannot be provided by real food in the hours following your ride. Indeed, a chocolate milk or a milk-based smoothie with a handful of frozen berries or half a banana followed by some dried fruit or nuts can perform a pretty similar job if you're in a hurry. If you are going to use a supplement, I'd go for whey protein, which is digested quickly, but you only need a single scoop in a smoothie or shake.

Many manufacturers play on the myth that you need to consume it more or less as soon as you're off the bike, but this is really your choice.

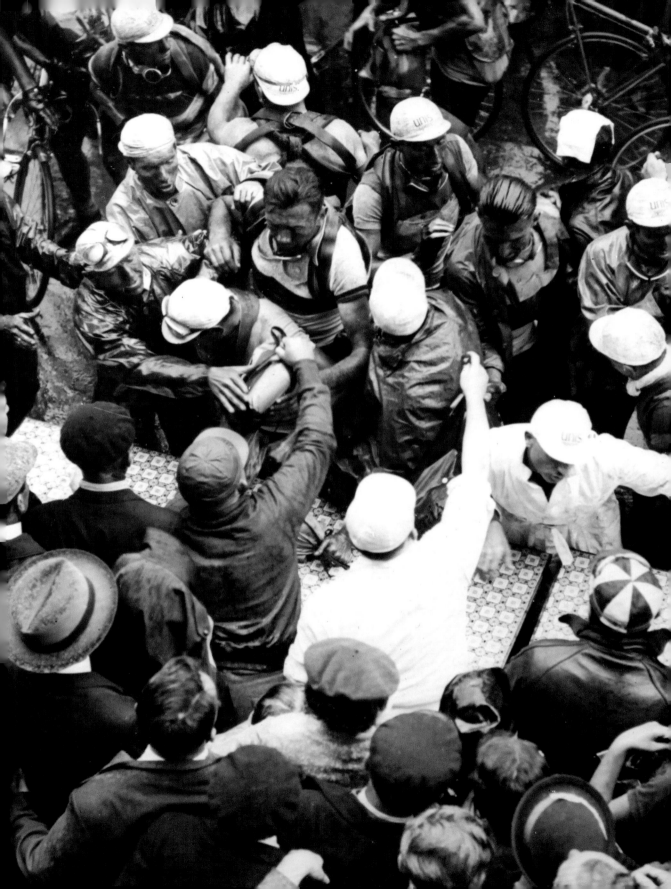

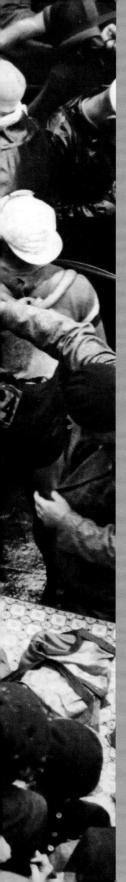

Feeding station frenzy! In the early days of racing, riders would raid bars and cafes for food. Formal feed stations were introduced in 1919, but riders still had to stop to collect food from the tables. Those who grab and go quickest saved the most time.

PROTEIN PUNCHEURS

After a punishing ride, your muscles will need some TLC. Chicken, fish, eggs and even chickpeas all rate highly for protein, so get them onside. In this section you'll find my slightly twisted versions of chicken nuggets (I call them Chicken Murch-nuggets – see page 110) and a Fish finger sarnie (see page 123), but then I'm all for experimentation. Nuts top the protein rankings, too, so why not try mixing equal quantities of DIY nut butter (see page 112) with sweet chilli sauce and soy sauce, then add to grated carrot for an awesome salad base or serve with teriyaki chicken or grilled salmon and some steamed rice.

FREI-SPEED FALAFELS

These high-protein lovelies are a race-week favourite of the small and mighty vegetarian, mountain bike world champion and Olympic medallist, Sina Frei.

I bake them as a healthier option and they can be eaten hot or cold. This recipe makes plenty, as they're quite tricky to do in small portions, so feel free to freeze or share.

Makes 12

480 g (1 lb 1 oz) cooked chickpeas

4 garlic cloves, finely chopped

40 g (1½ oz) fresh coriander

30 g (1¼ oz) fresh parsley

zest of 1 lemon

2 teaspoons ground coriander

2 teaspoons ground cumin

2 teaspoons smoked paprika

1 teaspoon BBQ spice

100 ml (½ cup) extra virgin olive oil

3 tablespoons gram flour

salt and pepper

Tahini dressing

250 g (9 oz) Greek yoghurt

juice of 1 lemon

1 tablespoon tahini

2 tablespoons fresh mint, chopped

pinch of smoked paprika

2 tablespoons extra virgin olive oil

salt and pepper

1. Preheat the oven to 180°C/350°F/Gas 5.

2. Blend all the ingredients, with the exception of the olive oil, gram flour and seasoning, together in a food processor.

3. Gradually add the olive oil and then incorporate the gram flour. Season well.

4. Shape into 12 balls, although there's nothing that says a falafel has to be round, so make them into squares if you want to. Place on a baking tray and bake for 35 minutes. Alternatively, you can cook these in an air fryer at 160°C/320°F for 12 minutes.

5. To make the dressing, whisk together all the ingredients and adjust the seasoning. For a slightly more substantial snack or even what you might describe as a meal, stuff the falafels and dressing into a toasted pitta bread along with some salad.

Nutrition per serving:
Energy: 199 kcal | Total carbohydrate: 9.8 g (of which sugars: 1.2 g)
Fat: 14 g | Fibre: 3.3 g | Protein: 6.8 g | Salt: 0.04 g

FLYING SCOTSMAN SARDINES

This Asian take on sardines on toast is a homage to the man, the myth, the great innovator that is Graeme Obree.

Graeme was inventive in his riding positions and bike building, but he likes his food straight, from rolled balls of marzipan on the bike to a 'jam piece' (jam sandwich) for fuelling and, famously, sardines on toast as a recovery meal. A couple of fried eggs will take this up a notch, or go full Obree and have yourself a large glass of full fat milk as well.

Serves 1

125 g (4 oz) tinned sardines in oil

1 teaspoon sriracha mayonnaise

salt and pepper

80–100 g (3–3$\frac{1}{2}$ oz) kimchi, either shop-bought or see recipe in *The Cycling Chef: Recipes for Getting Lean and Fuelling the Machine*

2 slices good quality bread

1. Remove any larger bones from the sardines.
2. Mix the sardines with the sriracha, and season with the salt and pepper.
3. Toast the bread, spoon on the kimchi and top with the sardine mix.
4. Go take your washing machine apart for bike parts…

Nutrition per serving:
Energy: 515 kcal | Total carbohydrate: 39 g (of which sugars: 5.2 g)
Fat: 21 g | Fibre: 6.2 g | Protein: 38 g | Salt: 3.7 g

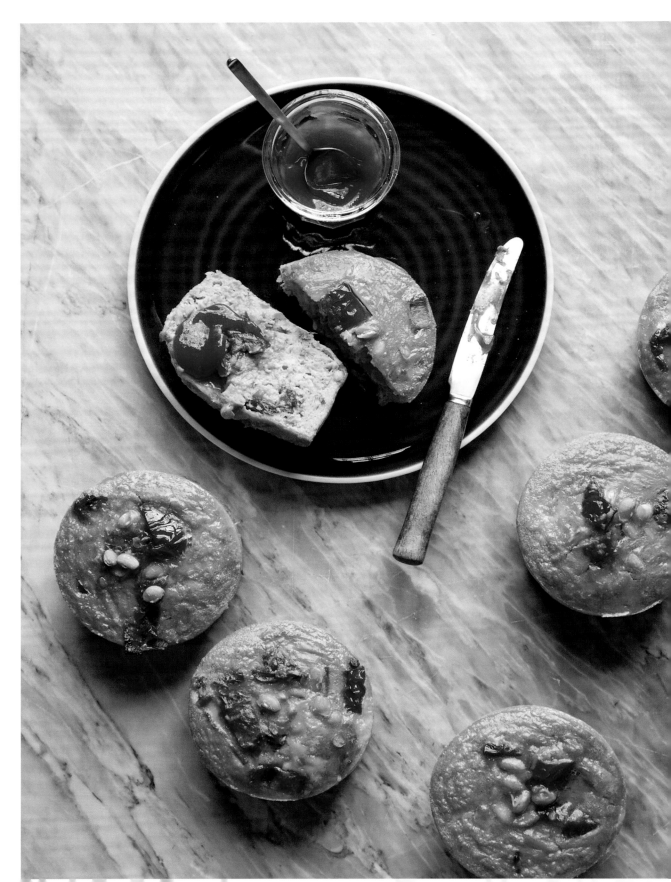

FULL ENGLISH FRITTATAS

There are few things finer than a breakfast-fry up – especially one that prepares you for a day in the saddle.

Grilling the bacon and using lean chicken sausages creates a healthy, protein-packed frittata, while blending the beans gives the eggs some structure and takes the protein levels up a notch.

Makes 6

4 rashers smoked back bacon

6 chicken sausages

235 g (8 ½ oz) cooked haricot blanc beans

2 teaspoons tomato purée

12 medium eggs

60 g (2 ½ oz) sun-dried tomatoes, roughly chopped

Nutrition per serving:

Energy: 178 kcal | Total carbohydrate: 4.4 g (of which sugars: 0.6 g)
Fat: 11 g | Fibre: 1.8 g | Protein: 15 g | Salt: 1.1 g

1. Preheat the oven to 130°C/250°F/Gas ½ and grease six 9 x 5 cm (3½ x 2 in) non-stick moulds.

2. Grill the bacon and chicken sausages until cooked. Set them aside and, when cool, finely slice the bacon and cut the sausages into chunks.

3. Blitz the cooked haricot beans with the tomato purée until smooth and transfer to a bowl.

4. Whisk in the eggs and season well.

5. Evenly distribute the bacon, sausages and sun-dried tomato between the moulds.

6. Half-fill the moulds with the egg mixture. Stir to ensure even distribution and then top up with the egg mix.

7. Place the moulds in the oven and cook for 35–40 minutes, but it's really important the oven isn't too hot, because if it is the egg mix will soufflé and go granular.

8. When they've cooled a little, remove the frittatas from the moulds. They can be stored in the fridge for two or three days. A nice way to reheat them is to cut them in half and pan-fry until golden or just pop them in the oven at 160°C/325°F/Gas 3 for 12 minutes.

Make a meal of it

Baked beans, sautéed mushrooms and a couple of slices of buttered toast... mug of tea. Sorted.

CHICKEN MURCH-NUGGETS

It's dirty secret time – and you must now swear a culinary omertà – my favourite post-race treat is fried chicken from a famous burger chain.

This version of that fast food classic is a familiar, but way-healthier, protein-packed dish which just might quash that desire to visit the takeaway on your way home.

Serves 2 (or one hungry Alan)

1 teaspoon smoked paprika

1 teaspoon Old Bay Seasoning or BBQ spice

1 teaspoon zaatar

1 teaspoon garlic powder

100 g (3½ oz) full fat Greek yoghurt

400 g (14 oz) chicken mini fillets

100 g (3½ oz) cornflakes

20 g (¾ oz) panko breadcrumbs or desiccated coconut

1 teaspoon smoked paprika

1 teaspoon BBQ spice

1 teaspoon sea salt flakes

Nutrition per serving:

Energy: 523 kcal | Total carbohydrate: 51 g (of which sugars: 17 g)

Fat: 8.2 g | Fibre: 4.8 g | Protein: 59 g | Salt: 4.2 g

1. Preheat the oven to 200°C/390°F/Gas 6.

2. Mix the first lot of spices and the yoghurt together, then mix in the chicken fillets.

3. Crush the cornflakes and panko breadcrumbs, keeping some texture. Stir in the smoked paprika, BBQ spice and salt.

4. Dip the chicken, one fillet at a time, into the cornflake mix and then place on a non-stick baking tray or the air fryer tray.

5. Bake at 200°C/390°F/Gas 6 for 22 minutes or cook in an air fryer, also at 200°C/390°F for 22 minutes. Serve with ketchup, BBQ or sweet chilli sauce.

Make a meal of it

Sweet potato oven fries and a large green salad. Or load up a large baguette and stack it with nuggets, salad and mayo or BBQ sauce.

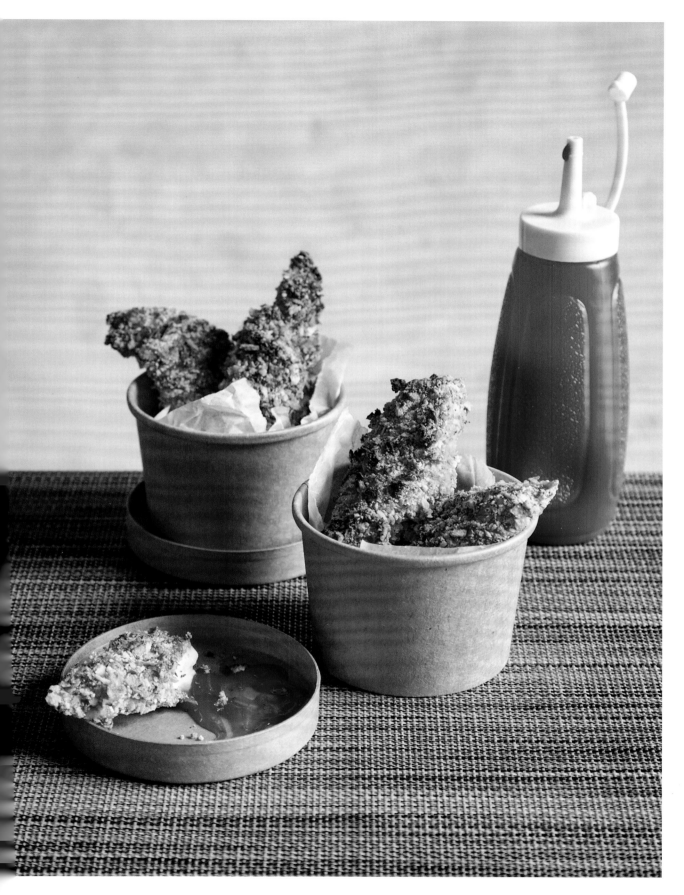

DIY NUT BUTTER

Nut butter has so many uses. It's ideal in sandwiches, wraps or on crispy rice cakes, as well as being an ingredient in a fair few recipes.

Making your own nut butter is an absolute no-brainer – simple and so much cheaper than any you'll buy in the shops. Peanuts work as well as anything, but avoid nuts with ridges, like pecans or walnuts, to avoid any potential contamination issues. Go on, give it a crack. I promise you will never buy the overpriced stuff again.

Makes 30 servings of 1 tablespoon

500 g (1 lb 2 oz) peanuts/macadamia/almond/cashew

Optional flavourings

1 tablespoon nut butter is a serving and for 100 g (3½ oz) nut butter add any of the following options:

good pinch of smoked salt flakes

1 teaspoon vanilla extract and 1 teaspoon cinnamon

2 tablespoons maple syrup

2 teaspoons red miso paste

1 teaspoon harissa

2 teaspoons Marmite

1. Lightly roast your nuts for 5–10 minutes to give them minimal colour.

2. Place them into a blender for 12–15 minutes until the desired texture has been achieved.

3. Store in a sealed jar in a cool place.

Nutrition per serving:
Energy: 101 kcal | Total carbohydrate: 1.8 g (of which sugars: 0.9 g) | Fat: 8.2 g | Fibre: 1 g | Protein: 4.5 g | Salt: 0.2 g

CHEEKY CHICKEN DOWSETT STYLE

This is peri-peri Portuguese-style chicken in honour of former hour record-holder Alex Dowsett's favourite post-race treat – and once cool, these spicy thighs are easily packable for the road.

When he is in the UK Alex loves a Nando's and their grilled chicken is actually pretty good for you. Just be careful on the sides, as coleslaw and fries can take this meal over to the dark side.

Serves 2

450 g (1 lb) boneless, skinless chicken thighs

Marinade

2 teaspoons smoked paprika

2 teaspoons garlic granules or powder

2 teaspoons dried chipotle chilli flakes

2 tablespoons dried parley

2 teaspoons dried oregano

2 teaspoons sea salt flakes

2 tablespoons olive oil

zest and juice of 1 lemon

zest and juice of 1 lime

1. Preheat the oven to 210°C/410°F/Gas 6.
2. Mix all the marinade ingredients together in an ovenproof dish. Add the chicken and rub well. Refrigerate and allow the chicken to marinade for, if possible, four hours.
3. Place chicken the oven for 25 minutes then finish under a hot grill for that authentic BBQ flavour.

Make a meal of it

Baked potato and some healthy vegetable slaw or chunky oven fries and corn on the cob. Señor Dowsett almost always would have had tomato ketchup on the side! Can't hide class.

Nutrition per serving:

Energy: 549 kcal | Total carbohydrate: 0.8 g (of which sugars: 0.8 g)

Fat: 34 g | Fibre: 1.6 g | Protein: 58 g | Salt: 5.2 g

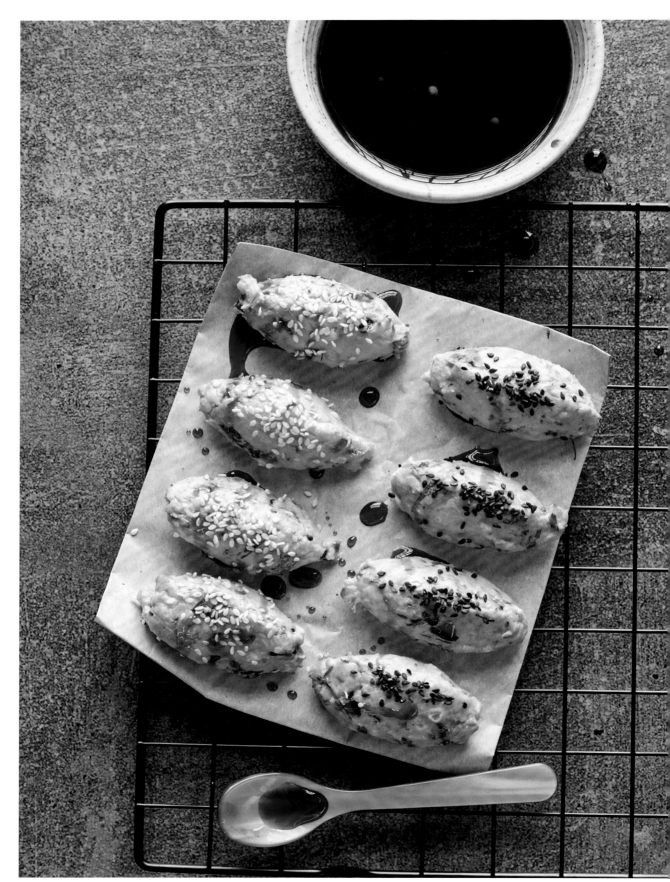

SALMON SESAME DIPPERS

This great little protein snack is also super-healthy. Salmon is a recovery food from the gods.

Not only does it give you a generous protein boost, but it's also rich in omega 3, which can increase blood flow to the muscles and replace lost minerals like potassium. You can also take the same approach to chicken if you fancy a meat-based dipper. Time to get dipping!

Makes 2 servings

220 g (7¾ oz) salmon fillet

1 large egg

170 g (6 oz) cooked potato

1 tablespoon corn flour

1 teaspoon salt

1 small red onion, finely diced

2 teaspoons green chilli, finely diced

1 tablespoon fresh coriander, chopped

zest of 1 lemon

pinch of Old Bay Seasoning

2 teaspoons of mixed sesame seeds

Dipping sauce

75 ml (4½ tablespoons) soy sauce

25 g (1 oz) honey

75 g (3 oz) sweet chilli sauce

100 g (3½ oz) ketjap manis (Indonesian sweet soy sauce)

1. Preheat the oven to 180°C/350°F/Gas 5.
2. Blend the salmon and egg in a food processor until you have a smooth paste.
3. Add the cooked potato, corn flour and salt. Pulse until well incorporated, but don't overwork.
4. Stir in the onion, chilli, coriander, lemon zest and spices.
5. Take a dessert spoon-sized dollop of the mixture – about 55 g (2¼ oz) – and form into a nugget. Place on a non-stick baking tray or an air fryer tray. Repeat.
6. Sprinkle the sesame seeds over the dippers.
7. Bake at 180°C/350°F/Gas 5 for 12 minutes or cook in an air fryer at 160°C/325°F for 10 minutes.
8. To make the dipping sauce, simmer all the ingredients together gently for 5 minutes.

Make a meal of it

Serve with a watercress or rocket salad and diced cucumber. Also works well with stir-fried rice noodles using the dipping sauce as a noodle dressing.

Nutrition per serving:
Energy: 545 kcal | Total carbohydrate: 53 g (of which sugars: 26 g)
Fat: 22 g | Fibre: 3.4 g | Protein: 32 g | Salt: 6.5 g

OLD BAY BAKED POTATO CAKES

Carbs 'n' protein in a very simple form are given some extra zip here with some of my favourite Cajun-style seasoning.

This base mix is easy to make and can be adapted to your own taste with feta, spring onions, cooked bacon, roasted red peppers or whatever. Just remember to turn the oven down for the second bake.

Makes 6

1.2 kg (2½ lbs) small baking potatoes

30 g (1¼ oz) olive oil

1 teaspoon smoked paprika

1 teaspoon Old Bay Seasoning

1 teaspoon salt

12 medium eggs

1 teaspoon smoked paprika

1 teaspoon Old Bay Seasoning

2 tablespoons tomato purée

Nutrition per serving:

Energy: 416 kcal | Total carbohydrate: 45 g (of which sugars: 4.3 g)

Fat: 16 g | Fibre: 6.1 g | Protein: 20 g | Salt: 1.8 g

1. Preheat the oven to 190°C/375°F/Gas 5 and grease six 9 x 5 cm (3½ x 2 in) non-stick moulds.

2. Place the potatoes, oil, paprika, Old Bay Seasoning and salt in a bowl and mix well.

3. Transfer the potatoes to a non-stick baking tray and bake them for 60–70 minutes, until they're soft.

4. Remove them from the oven, allow them to cool for 10 minutes, scoop out the flesh and set aside.

5. Shred the potato skins and put them back into the oven for 15 minutes.

6. Turn down the oven temperature to 130°C/250°F/Gas ½.

7. Allow the potato flesh and skins to cool down slightly.

8. Whisk the eggs and add the second lot of the paprika, Old Bay Seasoning and the tomato purée.

9. Whisk in the potato flesh and skin, making sure you keep the mix chunky.

10. Ladle the mix into the moulds, and sprinkle more smoked paprika and Old Bay on the top.

11. Bake again at the lower temperature for 40 minutes until firm to the touch.

12. Allow to cool for 10 minutes before removing from the moulds. To reheat, cut in half and sauté in butter for 4–5 minutes over a medium heat or pop them back in the oven for 10 minutes.

Make a meal of it

Large tomato salad with crushed avocado and black olives. Side of smoked salmon or grilled asparagus. Or bin off the salad and have baked beans!

CHAMP'S CHORIZO TOAST

Australian time-trial specialist Rohan Dennis responds well to the heavy training volume ahead of those big races.

This 'Aussie' (rather than French) toast is a great post-ride recovery dish. However, fatigue can affect the appetite for nutritionally dense food, yet I defy anyone to not want to eat when you smell that smoky sausage cooking.

Serves 2

100 g (3½ oz) smoked chorizo, sliced

1 tablespoon extra virgin olive oil, Spanish if you can

1 tablespoon honey

4 medium eggs

100 ml (½ cup) full fat milk

good pinch of smoked paprika

black pepper and sea salt flakes

4 thick slices sourdough bread

Nutrition per serving (2 slices):
Energy: 716 kcal | Total carbohydrate: 57 g (of which sugars: 14 g)
Fat: 37 g | Fibre: 3.4 g | Protein: 38 g | Salt: 3.2 g

1. Cook the chorizo in the oil in a large sauté pan over a medium heat until it's nicely coloured.

2. Remove it from the pan (don't wash the pan) and place it in an ovenproof dish. Drizzle over the honey and place in a warm oven to 'hold'.

3. Whisk the eggs with the milk, paprika and some seasoning.

4. Soak the sourdough in the egg mix.

5. Put the chorizo pan back on to a medium heat – you want the chorizo oil to cook the eggy bread in.

6. Shake off any excess egg and cook the bread for 2 minutes on each side until golden brown.

7. To serve, place the chorizo on top of the golden eggy toast and spoon over the honey juices.

Make a meal of it

You could make it a bit more substantial with crushed avocado and a large green salad.

CRISPY FRIED ASIAN-STYLE EGGS

Over-easy or sunny side up, who doesn't like a fried egg? Eggs are little protein bombs and great for recovery – but can seem a little bland.

This dish ramps up the taste with some zinging Asian flavours. It uses ketjap manis, a thick, syrupy, quite sweet soy sauce from Indonesia, and silky and rich sriracha mayo for a great South East Asian kick.

Serves 1

2 medium eggs

1 tablespoon olive oil

14 g ($\frac{1}{2}$ oz) sweet chilli sauce

10 g ketjap manis

10 g soy sauce

1 spring onion, finely chopped

dash of sriracha mayonnaise

pinch of sesame seeds

pinch of crispy onions

Nutrition per serving:

Energy: 315 kcal | Total carbohydrate: 10 g (of which sugars: 7.9 g)
Fat: 23 g | Fibre: 0 g | Protein: 17 g | Salt: 3.2 g

1. Heat the oil in a large non-stick pan over a medium heat.
2. Crack in the eggs and cook them for 2 minutes each side until nicely coloured.
3. Mix the sweet chilli sauce, ketjap manis and soy sauce together.
4. Pour over the eggs and cook for a further minute until nicely glazed.
5. Freestyle the spring onion, sriracha, sesame and crispy onions over the top.

Make a meal of it

Absolute simple banger, served with cooked basmati rice. Add extra sriracha to the rice. Or pop the eggs in soft bread rolls for a spicy bap.

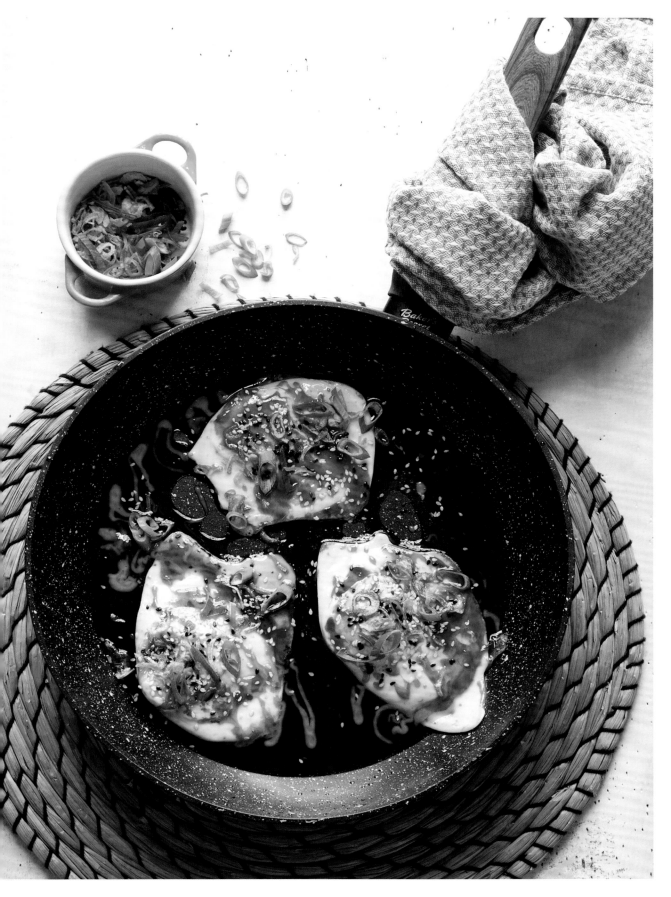

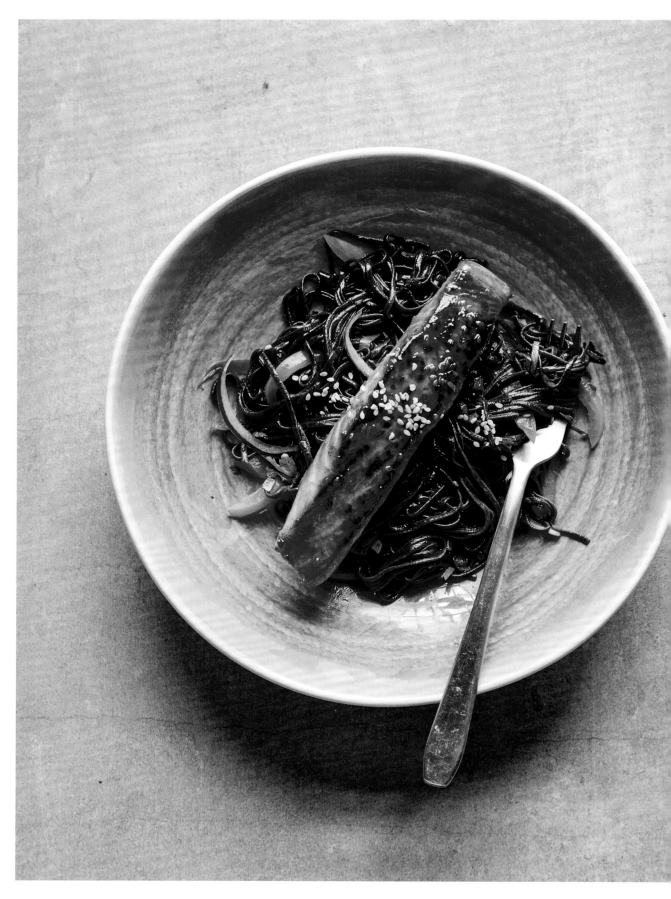

MISO SESAME SALMON

Teriyaki sauce is an instant life-saver and an absolute banger – it just works.

Cook the salmon (or smoked tofu or white firm fish) in the sauce with the veg, then mix with carbs of your choice – black rice noodles look the bomb.

Serves 2

150 g (5 oz) teriyaki sauce

2 teaspoons red miso paste

2 teaspoons toasted sesame oil

zest and juice of 1 lime

2 x 150 g (5 oz) salmon fillets

1 red pepper, finely sliced

1 medium red onion, finely sliced

salt and pepper

1 teaspoon sesame seeds

2 tablespoons fresh coriander, chopped

Nutrition per serving:

Energy: 496 kcal | Total carbohydrate: 18 g (of which sugars: 16 g)
Fat: 29 g | Fibre: 3.2 g | Protein: 38 g | Salt: 8.9 g

1. Preheat the oven to 150°C/300°F/Gas 2.

2. Mix the teriyaki sauce with the red miso paste, sesame oil and lime.

3. Place the salmon into the mix and marinade for 30 minutes.

4. Mix the pepper and onion together, season and place in a small ovenproof dish.

5. Place the salmon on top of the veg and pour over any excess marinade.

6. Bake for 15 minutes, then sprinkle on the sesame seeds and coriander. Eat hot or cold.

Make a meal of it

Serve with 100g per person of noodles or HB sauce (see page 89) with an Asian veg mix.

TUNA 'MAYONNAISE' CUCUMBER SUSHI

A sushi cheat that is simple to make, this looks the business and still packs a fresh-tasting protein and carb boost.

The thing that makes it is the thinking bike-rider's ketchup – sriracha mayo. Source fresh tuna if you can, but if that's not available you can also use fresh or smoked salmon. These can easily be wrapped for ride food on cooler days.

Serves 2

1 large cucumber

240 g (9 oz) fresh tuna

$\frac{1}{2}$ red onion, very finely diced

2 small spring onions, finely sliced

2 tablespoons sriracha mayonnaise

salt and pepper

120 g (4 oz) cooked and seasoned sushi rice

1 teaspoon black sesame seeds

1 teaspoon white sesame seeds

50 g (2 oz) crispy fried shallots

1. Cut your cucumber into three, then cut each piece in half horizontally and slice a small amount of the outer skin off to make a flat, stable surface. Scoop out the seeds with a small teaspoon, dry with some kitchen paper and set aside. They should look like mini cucumber boats!

2. Finely dice the fresh tuna, and mix it with the red onion, spring onion and sriracha. Adjust the seasoning and set aside.

3. Fill the 'channel' in the cucumber with the sushi rice, top with the tuna mayo and then sprinkle on the sesame seeds and crispy onions in an arty fashion.

Nutrition per serving:
Energy: 483 kcal | Total carbohydrate: 39 g (of which sugars: 12 g)
Fat: 19 g | Fibre: 4.2 g | Protein: 38 g | Salt: 1.1 g

FISH FINGER SARNIE

This is comfort food at its finest, made easy with some old-school chef flavours and techniques.

Who needs a gastro pub version when you can knock this up at home with next to no trouble? You can also make up a healthy tartare sauce, but no stress if you want to use mayo instead of crème fraîche.

Serves 2

250 g (9 oz) haddock fillet

2 tablespoons plain flour

pinch of cayenne pepper

1 teaspoon garlic powder

1 teaspoon turmeric

3 eggs

75 ml (4½ tablespoons) milk

120 g (4 oz) panko breadcrumbs or crushed cornflakes or a 50/50 mix

olive oil

4 slices soft white bread

Easy tartare sauce

2 tablespoons low fat crème fraîche

1 tablespoon gherkins, chopped

1 tablespoon capers, chopped

2 tablespoons parsley, chopped

zest of 1 lemon

few drops lemon juice

salt and pepper

1. Preheat the oven to 190°C/375°F/Gas 5.
2. Cut the haddock into even 'fingers' about 8 x 3 cm (3 x 1 in) in size.
3. Mix the flour with the cayenne, garlic powder and turmeric and set aside.
4. Whisk the eggs with the milk and set aside.
5. Place the breadcrumbs in a tray.
6. Take a piece of fish and dip it into the flour, shaking off any excess. Then dip it into the egg, shaking off any excess again. Finally, roll it in the breadcrumbs, ensuring it is evenly covered, and place on a non-stick baking tray. Repeat this process until all the fish done.
7. Spray with olive oil and bake at 190°C/375°F/Gas 5 for 16 minutes or cook in an air fryer at 180°C/350°F for 12 minutes.
8. Make the tartare sauce by mixing all the ingredients together.
9. Spread a generous spoonful of tartare on a slice of bread, load up with fish fingers and top with another slice of bread to form a sandwich.

Nutrition per serving:
Energy: 782 kcal | Total carbohydrate: 88 g (of which sugars: 6.2 g)
Fat: 24 g | Fibre: 5.3 g | Protein: 51 g | Salt: 2.4 g

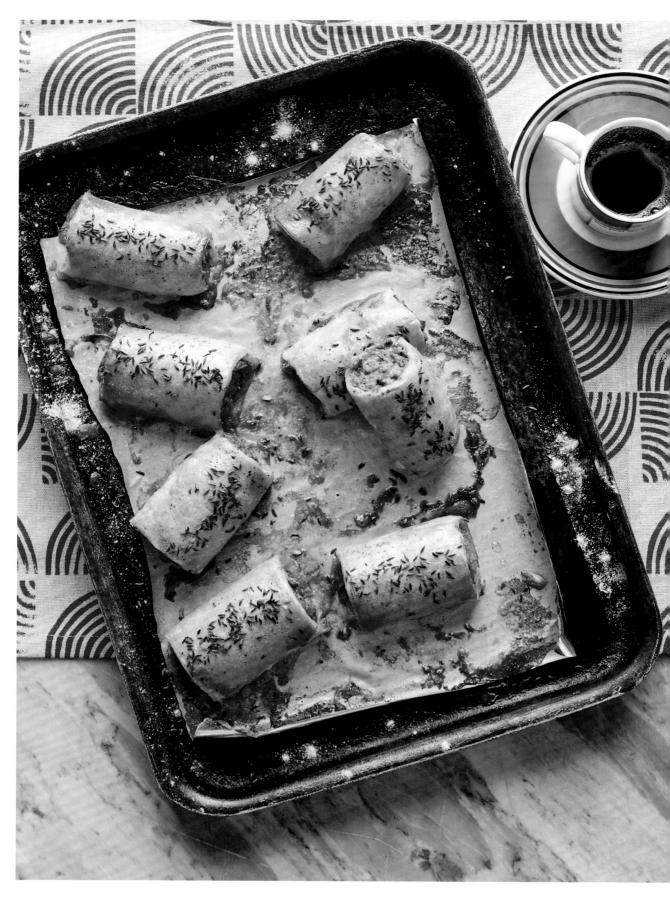

GREG'S REVENGE SAUSAGE ROLL

Tenuous title link ahead! Three times Tour de France winner Greg LeMond nearly died while shooting wild turkeys...

That said, if life is too short to make your own puff pastry, then maybe the same is true of holding grudges against turkeys. What's great about turkey thigh meat, though, is that it's low in fat and high in protein, and using ready-rolled pastry makes this an easy comfort food to make.

Makes 6

150 g (5 oz) smoked streaky bacon

2 teaspoons olive oil

2 teaspoons caraway seeds

3 teaspoons Dijon mustard

400 g (14 oz) turkey thigh mince

black pepper

280 g (10 oz) puff pastry, ready-rolled

1 egg yolk, beaten

extra pinch of caraway seeds

Nutrition per serving:
Energy: 355 kcal | Total carbohydrate: 17 g (of which sugars: 0.5 g)
Fat: 21 g | Fibre: 0.7 g | Protein: 23 g| Salt: 1.3 g

1. Preheat the oven to 200°C/390°F/Gas 6.

2. Finely chop the bacon, place in a non-stick pan with the olive oil and caraway seeds, and cook over a medium heat until it's golden brown and crispy.

3. Strain off the excess fat from the bacon with a sieve, then set it aside to cool.

4. Once cool, mix with the Dijon mustard, then stir into the turkey mince and season with black pepper.

5. Place a 10 cm x 12cm (4 x 5 in) piece of puff pastry onto a floured surface and divide the mince mix into six equal parts – each one should weigh about 75 g (3 oz).

6. Form each piece of mince into a sausage, place it on the pastry, brush one edge with the egg yolk so that the pastry binds, and fold the pastry over. For me it is best to have a lip on the pastry.

7. Place the rolls on to a non-stick tray, brush with egg yolk and sprinkle some caraway on top.

8. Bake for 18 minutes. Remove from the oven and place on a cooling rack for 10 minutes before eating.

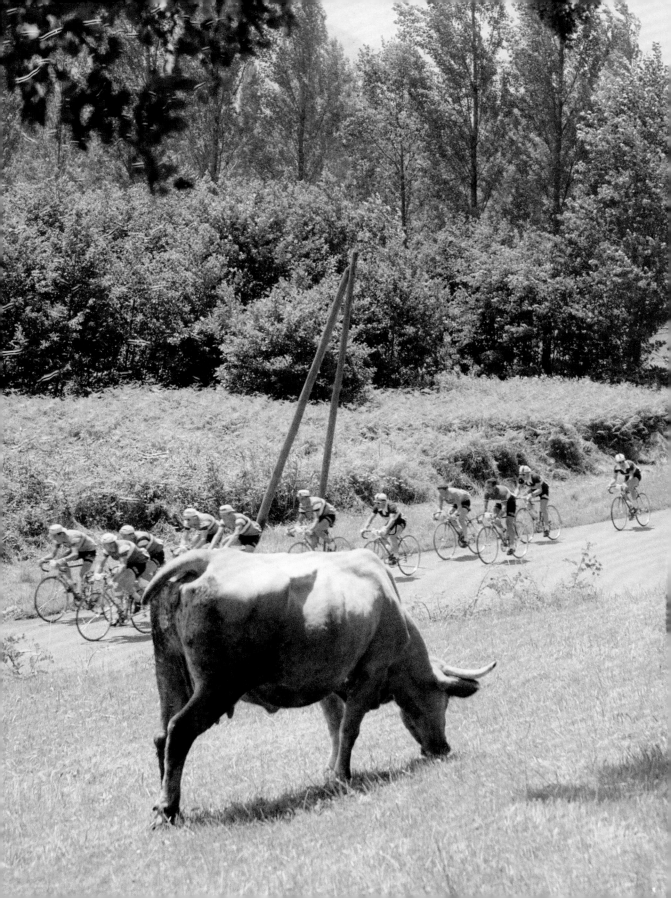

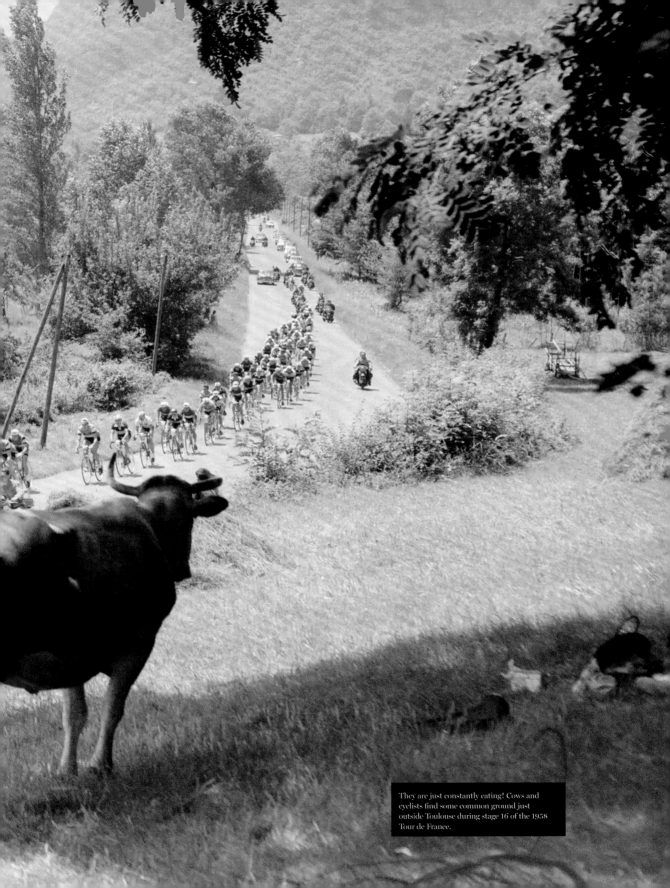

They are just constantly eating! Cows and cyclists find some common ground just outside Toulouse during stage 16 of the 1958 Tour de France.

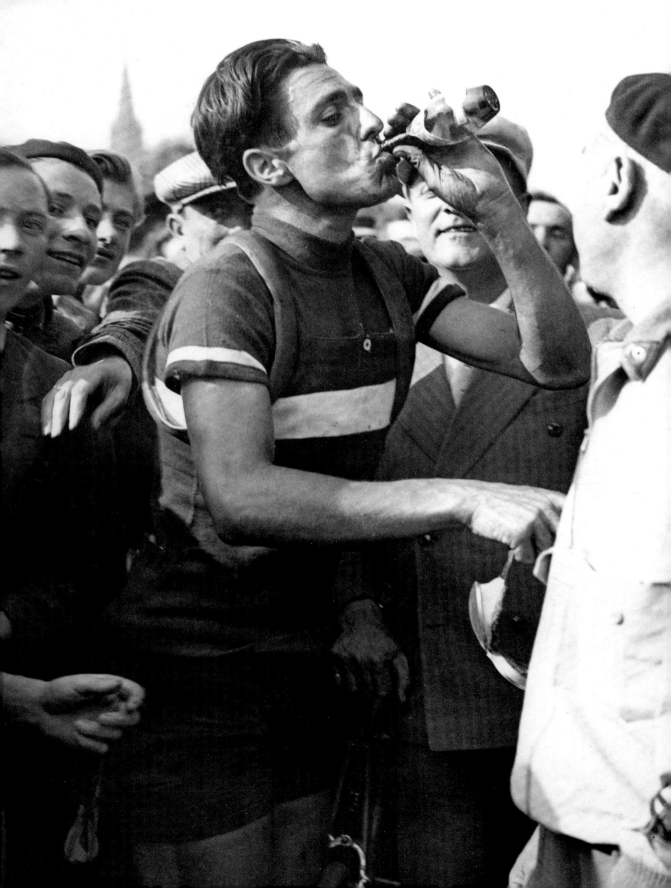

START RIGHT

Preparation for a tough day in the saddle doesn't start at breakfast. Satisfying the body's nutritional demands means playing the long game, adjusting levels of training, and ensuring we have the nutrients to stay fit and healthy. When a race day or a tough ride comes along, it doesn't mean you need to change your diet dramatically, but you do need to consider what you require to get the best out of your body.

The Swiss team have breakfast in Metz before the start of the 1951 Tour de France. Giovanni Rossi (far left) won the opening stage to Reims, while Hugo Koblet (near right) would go on to win the Tour.

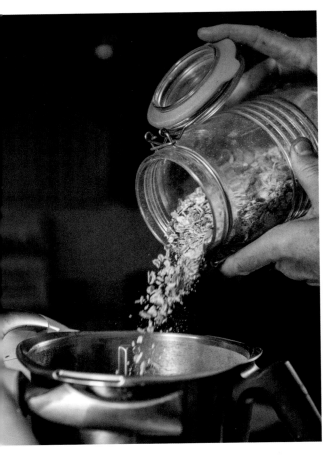

Enjoy your time in the kitchen. It's such a pleasure to cook with fresh and flavoursome ingredients.

Proper preparation before your ride should include your fuelling status as well as the state of your bike. The most important aspect on ride day is ensuring that your muscles' glycogen (energy) stores are well stocked. Glycogen is sourced from glucose, which is created by carbohydrates in the food you eat. It cannot be stored indefinitely. Normal everyday living will deplete most of your stores in a day or so and exercise or a low-carbohydrate diet will accelerate the rate at which it is lost.

Non-sporty people are recommended to consume 225 g to 325 g of carbohydrate a day and we can use this as a baseline for cyclists. If you are training two or three hours or more on most days of the week you will be looking to nearly double this to replenish your glycogen levels. As long as you do this, you will be in a good position to prepare for a particularly long or intense ride.

Carbo loading used to be a popular term for runners and cyclists preparing for endurance events. Based on the importance of glycogen levels at the start of a race, it had some scientific backing. However, the more complex scientific details were often disregarded and replaced by a general sense that it was fine to pile into as much pasta (and it was sometimes extended to pizza and pies) as possible on the eve of an event. The problem with this is that we can only store around 400 g of glycogen. Load too many carbs and it will just turn to fat.

Topping up your glycogen levels in the days running up to a big event is a much more sensible course of action. Add 10 per cent or so to your daily intake and bear in mind that not all your carbs need to come from rice and pasta. Fruit, vegetables, oats and beans are all nutrient-dense, fibre-rich and tasty options. By all means have a decent meal with plenty of carbs on the eve of a race, but don't overdo it – indigestion, bloating and other digestive discomfort will pose a far bigger problem. Like all aspects of fuelling, every individual's requirements differ, and will vary according to the intensity and duration of each session or race.

BEST MEAL OF THE DAY

Your morning meal is often your last chance to attend to your energy requirements before you get on the bike. While you're asleep you will not have depleted your muscles' glycogen levels very much, so how much topping up is required depends on how hard you have trained in the week and how heavily you have compensated in your diet. However, what will have reduced overnight is the glycogen stored in your blood and particularly in your liver. This is used to rejuvenate and repair cells, especially those in the brain. The liver can store around 100 g of glycogen, but it is possible that can reduce by 10 g an hour overnight.

You need to think about having your breakfast around three hours before the start of the ride... Now I've ridden long enough to know that cycle event and race organisers are no great respecters of the lie-in. Pulling on the leggings in the semi-darkness of morning is an occupational hazard and many of us just don't fancy tucking into a hefty breakfast in those early hours. We'll come to you later.

Taking breakfast two or three hours before your ride gives your digestive system plenty of time to do its work. You can include some fat and protein in your meal (important if you are on a stage race or have scant recovery time), and load up on foods with slow-release carbohydrates. This gives you a wide choice, from eggs on toast to cereal or a smoothie.

Non-sporty people are recommended to consume 225 g to 325 g of carbohydrate a day and we can use this as a baseline for cyclists.

The optimal time to drink coffee is around an hour before your ride, because that is how long it takes to reach its peak in the blood stream.

Then there is oatmeal, God's gift to cyclists. As bircher or warm porridge it has carbs, healthy fats and protein, and is high in soluble fibre, which slows digestion. You could even broaden your horizons and try cold meats, beans, vegetables, burritos or soup – they work for millions in countries around the world. Steer clear of anything too fatty, though. Unfortunately, we're looking longingly at you here, bacon – it takes too long to digest and will sit in your stomach for most of your ride before it can be used as energy.

A good breakfast isn't complete without a decent cup of coffee to wake you up. Your morning brew can do more than just that. It can facilitate the burning of fat rather than glycogen, stimulate the nervous system, thus making you more alert, and improve blood flow. The optimal time to drink coffee is around an hour before your ride, because that is how long it takes to reach its peak in the blood stream. However, go easy on the milk and avoid the full fat stuff as you may find it slows digestion.

It is worth being generally aware of your hydration levels before you get on the bike. Don't go mad as you can over-hydrate and you will find yourself wanting to pee pretty soon after setting off. A glass of water with your breakfast and, if necessary, before you leave the house should be enough.

The great thing about breakfast is that it can be prepared quickly or in advance. Oats can be soaking while you're sleeping, smoothies can be made the night before or whizzed up in seconds when you wake, and even scrambled eggs on toast is ready in a matter of minutes. However, if you are not able (or willing) to have an early breakfast, don't rush it. Just have less fat and protein, and more easily digested carbohydrates, and remember that the closer you get to the start of the ride, the less time your body has to digest food.

Around 90 minutes before you set off is the latest you should tuck into a substantial breakfast. If possible, now wait until 15 minutes or so before your ride begins. If you eat 90 minutes or more before exercise, your body has enough time to digest food; however any less and you will feel tired and sluggish as your blood glucose levels drop. Ideally, the levels will be rising or levelled off when you are on the bike.

At this point you are best sticking to small portions of carbohydrate-heavy food and avoiding fat and fibre as much as possible. A smoothie, a muffin, low-fat yoghurt and fruit or a piece of toast and jam are the kind of things to set you on your way. If all else fails and you have absolutely no time to grab a bit to eat, then a gel or an energy bar at the start line is your best option.

SLOW-RELEASE BREAKFASTS

For cyclists preparing for a big ride breakfast is mostly about the carbs. A little fat and protein can help stave off the hunger, but energy is the thing. The Glycaemic Index (GI) is an established ranking of foods that contain carbohydrates based on how slowly or quickly they are digested and increase blood glucose levels. As a rule of thumb, cyclists should look to low or moderate GI foods at breakfast to provide a slow release of energy during the ride.

Low GI Milk, yoghurt, grapes, apples, bananas, peanut butter (no added sugar), tortilla wraps, pasta, orange juice.

Moderate GI Wholegrain, granary or pitta bread, honey, muesli, pancakes, porridge oats, cranberry juice, dried fruit, low-sugared cereals (for example, Special K), ice cream, flapjacks.

High GI White bread, bagels, baguette, melon or watermelon, cranberries, biscuits, sugared cereals (for example, Cheerios), cereal bars, doughnuts, scones.

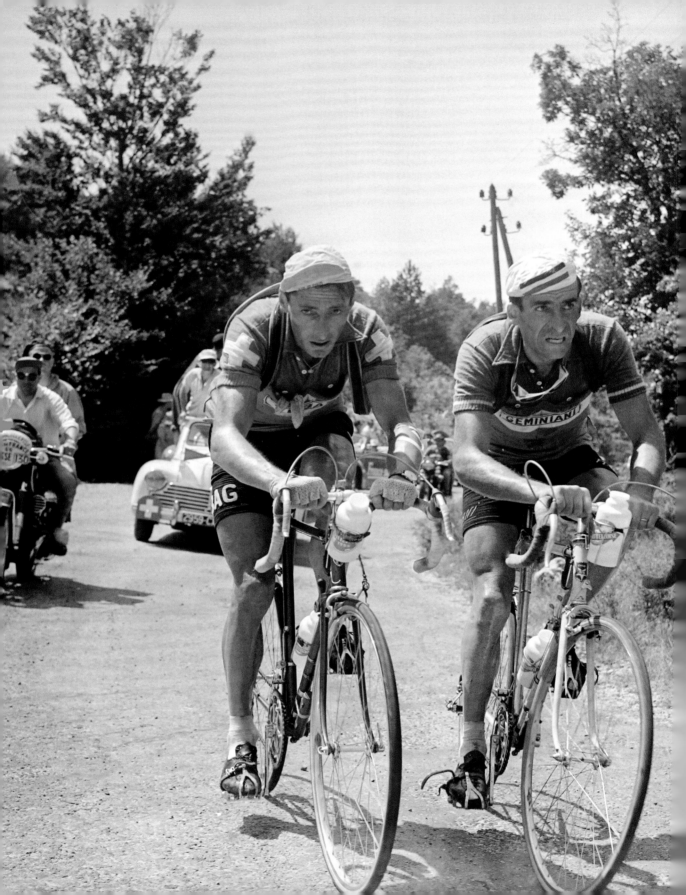

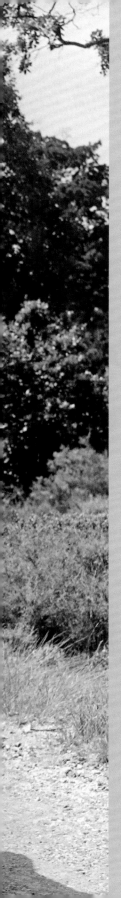

RECIPES

POST- AND PRE-RIDE EATS AND TREATS

Appetite fatigue and time deprivation are the enemies of the well-nourished cyclist. That ends here with a selection of impossible-to-ignore and easy-to-prepare recipes. There are the sweets – try a White chocolate miso blondie (see page 150). There are the snacks – I give you Go hard avo hummus (see page 155). And then there are simply uncategorisable dishes – check out the Salted caramel shortbreads… with black olive (see page 154) or my Jam soufflé breakfast dessert (see page 163) They are all designed to delight both before you hit the saddle and after you've earned your R&R. Enjoy!

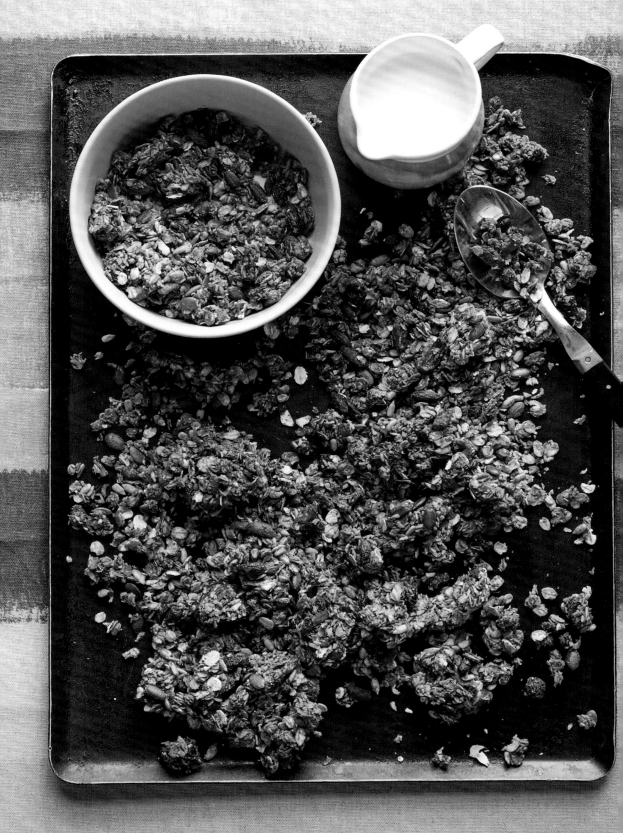

GO! GO! GO! GRANOLA

This high-carb, pre-ride breakfast is perfect if you're not really a morning person. All you have to do is pour it into a bowl and splash on your milk of choice.

It goes down well, is easy on the stomach and is packed with fast- and slow-releasing carbohydrates, protein, fibre, vitamins and minerals.

Makes 12 servings

75 g (3 oz) honey

75 g (3 oz) organic blackstrap molasses

55 g ($2\frac{1}{4}$ oz) coconut oil

250 g (9 oz) jumbo rolled oats

75 g (3 oz) desiccated coconut

75 g (3 oz) dates, chopped

60 g ($2\frac{1}{2}$ oz) pumpkin seeds

60 g ($2\frac{1}{2}$ oz) sunflower seeds

40 g ($1\frac{1}{2}$ oz) goji berries

40 g ($1\frac{1}{2}$ oz) golden raisins

2 teaspoons ground ginger

2 teaspoons ground cinnamon

$\frac{1}{2}$ teaspoon salt

1. Preheat the oven to 140°C/285°F/Gas 1 and line a baking tray with greaseproof paper.
2. Melt the honey, molasses and coconut oil together.
3. Place the dry ingredients in a large bowl. Stir the wet ingredients into the dry ingredients and mix thoroughly.
4. Spread out the mixture evenly on the lined tray.
5. Bake for 45 minutes, gently mixing with a fork every 15 minutes. The granola will still be sticky when it comes out of the oven, but will cool to a nice crispiness.
6. One serving weighs 68 g ($2\frac{1}{2}$ oz). Store in an airtight container for up to a week.

Nutrition per serving:

Energy: 300 kcal | Total carbohydrate: 33 g (of which sugars: 16 g)

Fat: 15 g | Fibre: 4.3 g | Protein: 6.4 g | Salt: 0.27 g

CHOCOLATEY CARDAMOM PROTEIN MUFFINS

Muffins are the time-poor cyclist's friend. Soft, sweet and perfect for nutritional purposes, grab one before you ride, or break into bite-sized pieces, wrap and pack, and take a couple with you on the bike.

This recipe is a complete chocolate fest, with the fruity, earthy cardamom adding a distinctive, intriguing flavour.

Makes 8

300 g (11 oz) extra ripe banana

400 ml (1½ cups) chocolate soya milk

1 whole medium egg

35 g (1¼ oz) cocoa powder

180 g (6 oz) self-raising flour

150 g (5 oz) chocolate protein powder

1 tablespoon baking powder

good pinch of cinnamon

seeds from 3 cardamom pods

pinch of ground cardamom

pinch of salt

75 g (3 oz) white choc chips

Nutrition per serving:

Energy: 300 kcal | Total carbohydrate: 37 g (of which sugars: 18 g)

Fat: 6.4 g | Fibre: 2.3 g | Protein: 23 g | Salt: 0.93 g

1. Preheat the oven to 180°C/350°F/Gas 5 and line eight muffin moulds.

2. Add the banana, chocolate milk and egg to the bowl of a food processor (you can literally do all this in a food processor) and blend.

3. Gradually add the cocoa powder, flour, protein powder, baking powder and cinnamon.

4. Crush the seeds from the cardamom with a pestle and mortar.

5. Stir in the ground seeds, ground cardamom, salt and choc chips.

6. Fill the lined muffin moulds and bake for 15–20 minutes.

7. Allow to cool. These muffins are best eaten fresh, although they can be stored in an airtight container for 2 days.

SPICED COFFEE BREAD 'N' BUTTER PUDDING BARS

An updated, pocket-friendly version of the classic dessert – there's sourdough bread and coffee, but still no escaping the sweet taste of nostalgia.

I like using seeded sourdough to give the bar a bit more structure, but you can use any bread you like. The espresso gives it a caffeine boost, and some extra protein in your ride food is no bad thing either.

Makes 12

200 g (7 oz) golden caster sugar, plus extra tablespoon for topping

160 ml ($\frac{2}{3}$ cup) full fat milk

250 ml (1 cup) extra thick double cream

100 ml ($\frac{1}{2}$ cup) espresso (4 x 21 g shots)

2 teaspoons vanilla extract

2 teaspoons cinnamon

1 teaspoon freshly ground nutmeg

3 eggs

2 egg yolks

100 g ($3\frac{1}{2}$ oz) unsalted butter

600 g ($1\frac{1}{4}$ lb) day-old sourdough bread (8 slices)

120 g (4 oz) chopped dried fruit – apricots, raisins, cherries

Nutrition per serving:

Energy: 415 kcal | Total carbohydrate: 47 g (of which sugars: 27 g)
Fat: 21 g | Fibre: 1.6 g | Protein: 8 g | Salt: 0.61 g

1. Preheat the oven to 170°C/340°F/Gas 4 and line a small deep baking tray. I use a 20 x 24 cm (8 x $9\frac{1}{2}$ in) tin and foil-backed greaseproof paper, which is easy to get out.

2. Place 60 g ($2\frac{1}{2}$ oz) of the sugar into a heavy-bottom saucepan. Gently heat until the sugar has melted and formed a sugary base on the bottom of the pan. This ensures the milk and cream don't stick to the bottom of the pan.

3. Place the milk, cream, espresso, vanilla extract and spices in the pan and heat until just simmering. Allow to cool for 5–10 minutes.

4. Whisk together the eggs, yolks and remaining sugar in a bowl. Whisk the milk, cream and spice mix into the eggs. Set aside.

5. Spread the butter evenly on both sides of the bread.

6. Build up your pudding, starting with a layer of bread, followed by the dried fruit. Ladle on half of the spiced coffee custard and top with another layer of buttered bread.

7. Pour over the remainder of the spicy egg custard mix and refrigerate for 60 minutes.

8. Sprinkle on the remaining sugar and bake for 45–50 minutes until the top is puffy and golden brown.

9. Now you have choices. You can get stuck in or you can leave it to cool for 90 minutes, then cover with a sheet of greaseproof paper, place a light weight on top to press it down and refrigerate overnight. The following day, cut into chunks or bars.

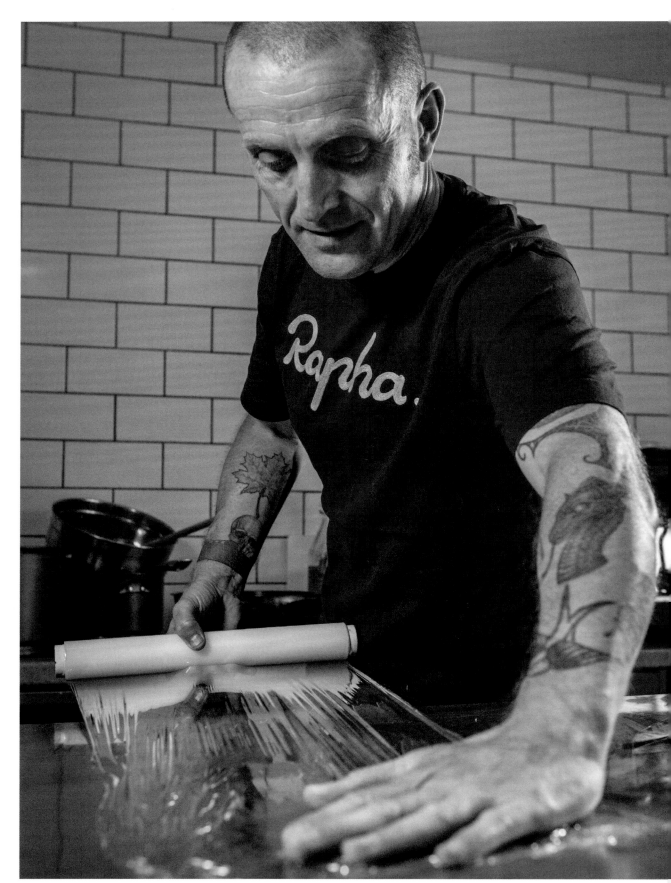

CHEWY OATMEAL RAISIN COOKIES

Sometimes just enjoying your food is enough – enter the cookie.
Sweet, chewy and with plenty of slow-release carbs to help ease
the guilt.

Oatmeal raisin cookies get a bad press, but this is often due to trying to make them too healthy. There is
plenty of goodness here along with the sweet hit, so get over yourself and enjoy this chewy cookie delight.

Makes 12

100 g ($3\frac{1}{2}$ oz) unsalted butter

185 g ($6\frac{1}{2}$ oz) sugar

1 egg

2 teaspoons vanilla extract

1 teaspoon baking powder

180 g (6 oz) gluten-free oats

140 g (5 oz) flour

100 g ($3\frac{1}{2}$ oz) raisins

75 g (3 oz) walnuts

Nutrition per serving:
Energy: 302 kcal | Total carbohydrate: 40 g (of which sugars: 22 g)
Fat: 13 g | Fibre: 2.5 g | Protein: 4.8 g | Salt: 0.04 g

1. Preheat the oven to 180°C/350°F/Gas 5 and line two baking trays.

2. Place the butter, sugar and egg in the bowl of a mixer and use the paddle attachment to mix them.

3. Add the vanilla, baking powder, oats, flour, raisins and walnuts, and mix until combined into a dough.

4. Refrigerate for an hour or so then divide into 12 equal balls.

5. Split between the baking trays and press each ball down slightly to form a thick disc. Allow space on the trays as the cookies will spread during cooking.

6. Bake for 10–12 minutes.

Cling film is brilliant for covering leftovers or wrapping food
items. Standard cling film, however, contains a PVC, an
unrecyclable plastic. Look for non-PVC or compostable film.

STICKY TOFFEE DATE MUFFINS

The super-versatile muffin is ready to take on any guise and as the sticky toffee pudding would one hundred per cent be one of my death row final meal choices, it's a nailed-on favourite.

This is one for when you think you're on your last legs – a muffin with a familiar taste and a to-die-for sweetness.

Makes 6

250 g (9 oz) ripe banana

100 g (3½ oz) brown sugar

100 g (3½ oz) dates, chopped

150 g (5 oz) butternut squash, grated

1 teaspoon ground ginger

1 teaspoon cinnamon

25 g (1 oz) black treacle

250 g (9 oz) plain flour

14g (½ oz) baking powder

25 g (1 oz) toasted coconut

2 medium eggs

3 tablespoons chocolate milk

1½ tablespoons olive oil

30 g (1¼ oz) fudge, cut into 6 chunks

30 g (1¼ oz) pecan nuts, chopped

1. Preheat the oven to 170°C/340°F/Gas 4 and grease six 9 x 5 cm (3½ x 2 in) non-stick moulds.

2. Place the banana, brown sugar, dates, butternut squash, ginger, cinnamon and treacle in the bowl of a mixer and use the paddle attachment to mix them.

3. Gradually add the flour, baking powder and toasted coconut.

4. Whisk the eggs, milk and olive oil together and add to the mixture.

5. Fill the moulds until just below the top.

6. Place a chunk of fudge in the centre of each muffin and sprinkle with the chopped pecans.

7. Bake for 25–30 minutes, checking the centre of the muffins with a small knife to ensure they are cooked.

8. Allow to cool and then remove from the moulds. Store at room temperature for up to 2 days.

Nutrition per serving:
Energy: 477 kcal | Total carbohydrate: 78 g (of which sugars: 44 g)
Fat: 13 g | Fibre: 4.7 g | Protein: 9.3 g | Salt: 0.83 g

MISO MARMITE PANCAKES

Umami! It's a great word, but not so easy to describe. We're talking about savoury deliciousness – and that's just what the combination of red miso paste and Marmite adds to these pancakes.

They can be used as a base or eaten on their own as a welcome change to sweet pancakes.

Makes 6

4 medium eggs

250 ml (1 cup) semi-skimmed milk

1 teaspoon Marmite

3 teaspoons red miso paste

250 g (9 oz) gluten-free self-raising flour

small bunch of spring onions, finely chopped

olive oil for frying

Nutrition per serving:
Energy: 270 kcal | Total carbohydrate: 34 g (of which sugars: 2.8 g)
Fat: 9.2 g | Fibre: 1.9 g | Protein: 11 g | Salt: 0.88 g

1. Whisk the eggs, milk, Marmite and miso paste together in a large bowl.

2. Gradually add the flour until you have a smooth batter.

3. Stir in the spring onions.

4. Heat a little oil in a non-stick pan. Pour in the batter using a 125 ml ($\frac{1}{2}$ cup) ladle so the pancakes are the same size. Cook for 60–90 seconds on each side, turning once.

5. This mix can be made up the day before, as pancake batter is often better the next day. You can also make smaller 'bite-size' pancakes.

WHITE CHOCOLATE MISO BLONDIES

This blondie pulls no punches on taste and nutrients, and has an irresistible combination of sweet and salty, with butter beans heading up the protein supply.

At last the blondie is the equal of its lauded dark chocolate rivals – yes, it really is that special.

Makes 12

80 g (3 oz) melted coconut oil

400 g (14 oz) butter beans, strained

130 g (4¼ oz) almond butter

140 g (5 oz) maple syrup

50 g (2 oz) white miso paste

2 medium eggs

160 g (5½ oz) gluten-free self-raising flour

pinch of salt

150 g (5 oz) frozen raspberries

60 g (2½ oz) desiccated coconut

75 g (3 oz) white chocolate chunks

50 g (2 oz) pecans

1. Preheat the oven to 180°C/350°F/Gas 5, and line and grease a 10 x 4 cm (4 x 1.5 in) rectangular mould (or any similar mould of your choice).

2. Blend the melted coconut oil, beans, almond butter, maple syrup, miso paste and eggs in a food processor to a smooth paste.

3. Add the flour and salt, and blend to a smooth batter.

4. Fold in the raspberries, coconut, white chocolate and pecans, reserving a few nuts for the top.

5. Spoon the mix into the mould, top with the reserved pecans and bake for 25 minutes until lightly brown on top and just set but still a bit wobbly.

6. Allow to cool and then store in the fridge.

Nutrition per serving:

Energy: 345 kcal | Total carbohydrate: 27 g (of which sugars: 13 g)

Fat: 22g | Fibre: 4.5 g | Protein: 8.4g | Salt: 0.68g

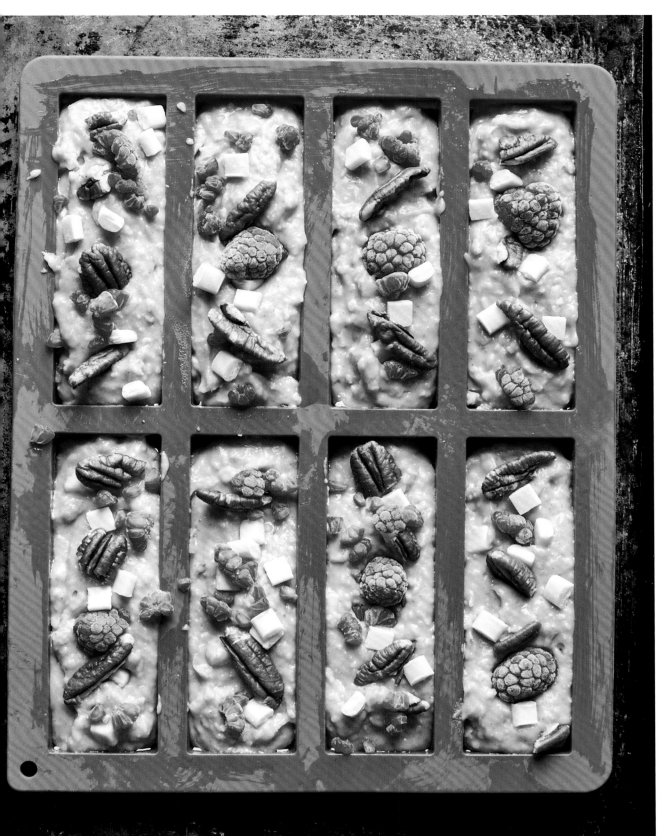

LAST LEGS ESPRESSO BROWNIE

Coffee and cycling – say no more. This brownie has a good shot of proper espresso in it to give you that kick just when you need it, plus it's a no-bake recipe which is really simple to prepare.

If you don't have an espresso machine at home, you can use a strong pod variety or good quality, strong instant coffee.

Makes 12

120 ml (4 oz) good quality espresso

300 g (11 oz) Deglet Noor dates

400 g (14 oz) black beans, strained

75 g (3 oz) Nutella

75 g (3 oz) nut butter

90 g ($3\frac{1}{2}$ oz) coconut oil, melted

70 g (3 oz) cocoa powder

60 g ($2\frac{1}{2}$ oz) cocoa nibs

60 g ($2\frac{1}{2}$ oz) bitter chocolate chips

Nutrition per serving:
Energy: 315 kcal | Total carbohydrate: 27 g (of which sugars: 23 g)
Fat: 19 g | Fibre: 5.3 g | Protein: 6.9 g | Salt: 0.2 g

1. Line a 20 x 20 cm (8 x 8 in) baking tray with greaseproof paper.

2. Make your strong coffee. If you're using an espresso machine, it should be the equivalent of three double espressos, extracted from 60 g ($2\frac{1}{2}$ oz) beans.

3. Pour the coffee on to the dates. I recommend the Deglet Noor variety of dates for this recipe, because they're drier and will soak up more coffee. Allow this mix to infuse and cool.

4. Place the black beans and coffee-soaked dates in a food processor and blend until smooth.

5. Add the Nutella, nut butter, coconut oil and coco nibs. Stir in the choc chips.

6. Press the mix firmly into the tray and refrigerate for 2 hours.

7. Cut into squares and store in an airtight container in the fridge.

CLANCY'S CLASSIC

Can you have too many brownie recipes? I very much doubt it. I'm a huge fan of incorporating pulses and veg into brownies for added protein, fibre and overall goodness.

Beetroot is a real performance-enhancer and this chocolate and beetroot brownie is a sure-fire winner, much like the man it's named after – Ed Clancy OBE, the most successful team pursuit cyclist in history.

Makes 12

300 g (11 oz) beetroot, cooked (not the stuff in vinegar)

100 g ($3\frac{1}{2}$ oz) unsalted butter

200 g (7 oz) 70 per cent chocolate

250 g (9 oz) Demerara sugar

3 medium eggs

1 teaspoon vanilla extract

pinch of salt

100 g ($3\frac{1}{2}$ oz) gluten-free plain flour

25 g (1 oz) cocoa powder

Nutrition per serving:

Energy: 310 kcal | Total carbohydrate: 35 g (of which sugars: 27 g)

Fat: 16 g | Fibre: 3 g | Protein: 5.3 g | Salt: 0.16 g

1. Preheat the oven to 180°C/350°F/Gas 5 and line a small baking tray with greaseproof paper.

2. Place the beetroot into a food processor and blend.

3. Melt the butter and chocolate together.

4. Add the butter and chocolate mix to the beetroot mix and blend until smooth.

5. Whisk the sugar, eggs and vanilla extract well until they double in volume.

6. Mix the beetroot choc mix and the eggs and sugar together.

7. Add the salt, flour and cocoa powder and mix until well incorporated.

8. Pour into the tray and bake for 20–25 minutes.

9. Allow to cool before cutting into 12 portions.

SALTED CARAMEL SHORTBREADS... WITH BLACK OLIVE

This is an on-the-bike version of an ace dessert I used to make back in the day when I was a fancy pants chef.

Remember, shortbread is a bit of an art, so don't overwork it and do allow the dough to sit in the fridge before rolling it out. The resulting biscuits are sweet, salty and crunchy.

Makes 12

Shortbread

300 g (11 oz) plain flour

200 g (7 oz) unsalted butter

100 g ($3\frac{1}{2}$ oz) caster sugar

Salted black olive caramel

200 g (7 oz) caramelised condensed milk

50 g (2 oz) finely diced Kalamata black olives

pinch of sea salt flakes

Homemade caramel

250 g (9 oz) caster sugar

40 g ($1\frac{1}{2}$ oz) liquid glucose

80 ml (5 tablespoons) whipping cream

1 teaspoon vanilla extract

200 g (7 oz) unsalted butter, diced

Nutrition per serving:

Energy: 310 kcal | Total carbohydrate: 36g (of which sugars: 18g)
Fat: 16g | Fibre: 1.1g | Protein: 3.9g | Salt: 0.34g

1. Preheat the oven to 170°C/340°F/Gas 4.

2. Place the flour, butter and sugar in a large bowl.

3. Work them together until they look like fine breadcrumbs.

4. Roll into a ball and refrigerate for 30 minutes. Trust me, this will make the shortbread easier to roll.

5. While the shortbread is relaxing somewhere cool, mix the caramel, olives and salt together. Taste this mix at least twice, adjust if necessary, then refrigerate it.

6. Roll out the shortbread on a flour-dusted worktop to a 5 mm ($\frac{1}{4}$ in) thickness. Cut into 5 cm (2 in) rounds and place carefully on a non-stick baking sheet. Refrigerate again for 15 minutes.

7. Sprinkle some additional sugar on top of the shortbread rounds and bake for 15 minutes until golden brown. Allow to cool on a cooling rack.

8. Before using caramel, taste it again just to make sure the flavour balance is right. Put 1 good teaspoon of the caramel mix onto the shortbread disc, top with another disc and set aside.

9. The shortbread will keep for a couple of days in an airtight container, but once you have added the caramel, make sure you eat them that day.

To make your own caramel

1. Place the sugar and glucose in a pan and cook over a medium or high heat until a nice caramel colour.

2. At the same time, place the cream and vanilla in a pan, warm them up, boil and then set aside.

3. Little by little, add the warm cream to the caramel base over a gentle heat.

4. Remove from the heat and gradually whisk in the butter. Allow to cool and firm up.

GO HARD AVO HUMMUS

Rich and super-creamy, this whizzed-up spread is ideal spread on wraps, toast or crispy rice crackers. It's a little bit like guacamole, a little bit like hummus and a lot like tasty.

But why the 'go hard'? Well, just take a look at the calories piling up here. You need to ride long and strong just to look at it.

Makes 6 servings

300 g (11 oz) avocado (2 medium avocados)

400 g (14 oz) chickpeas, strained

50 ml (3 tablespoons) lemon juice

150 ml ($\frac{2}{3}$ cup) olive oil

80 g (3 oz) tahini

small bunch of coriander

salt and pepper

2 tablespoons pumpkin seeds, toasted

1 teaspoon black sesame seeds

1. This is not rocket science – place everything in the food processor with exception of the seasoning and seeds. Blitz.

2. Season well, then sprinkle on those seeds.

Make a meal of it

This works so well as the basis of a large green salad. Serve with couscous, grilled asparagus and salmon.
It is also a perfect match with the Frei-speed falafels on page 106.

Nutrition per serving:
Energy: 465 kcal | Total carbohydrate: 7.3 g (of which sugars: 0.6 g)
Fat: 44 g | Fibre: 5.6 g | Protein: 7.9 g | Salt: 0.02 g

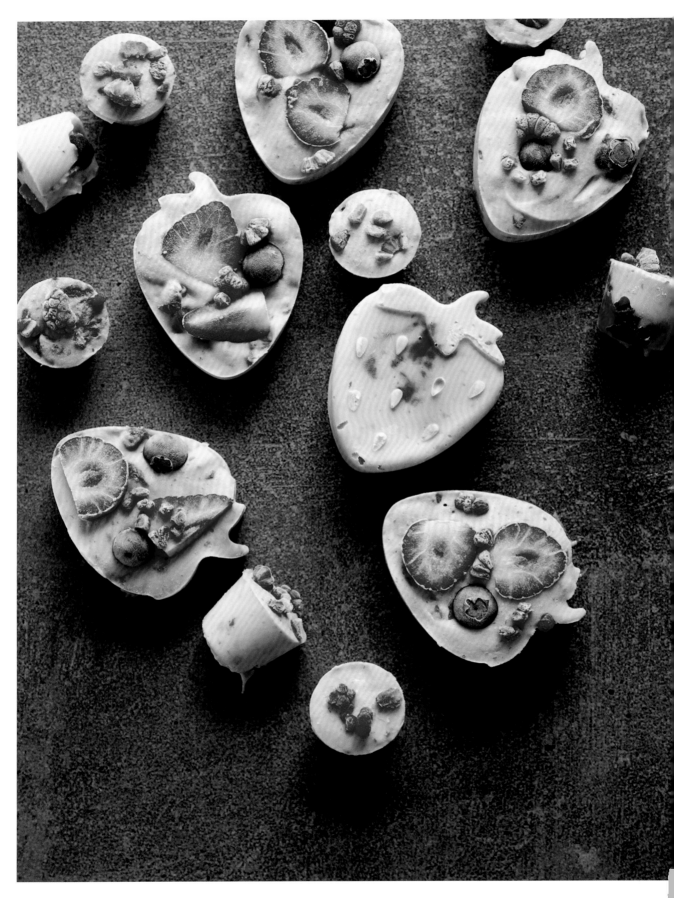

FROZEN YOGHURT PROTEIN BERRIES BITES

Recovery ice cream anyone? Well, near enough.

Pull one of these fruity and flavoursome guys out of the freezer after a long, hot ride and you can almost hear those muscles murmuring in appreciation.

Makes 12

500 g (1 lb 2 oz) full fat Greek yoghurt

200 ml ($\frac{3}{4}$ cup) almond milk

150 g (5 oz) vanilla protein powder

2 tablespoons good quality raspberry jam

60 g (2$\frac{1}{2}$ oz) runny honey

150 g (5 oz) frozen blueberries

150 g (5 oz) frozen raspberries or strawberries

100 g (3$\frac{1}{2}$ oz) white choc chips (optional)

Nutrition per serving:
Energy: 180 kcal | Total carbohydrate: 15 g (of which sugars: 14 g)
Fat: 6 g | Fibre: 1.4 g | Protein: 15 g | Salt: 0.22 g

1. Whisk together the yoghurt, almond milk and protein powder, ensuring there are no lumps.

2. Mix together the jam and honey.

3. Fold the frozen berries into the yoghurt, then add the jam. Don't overmix as you want a kind of raspberry ripple effect.

4. Pour into ice lolly or large ice cube moulds – use any shape you like – and freeze for at least 8 hours.

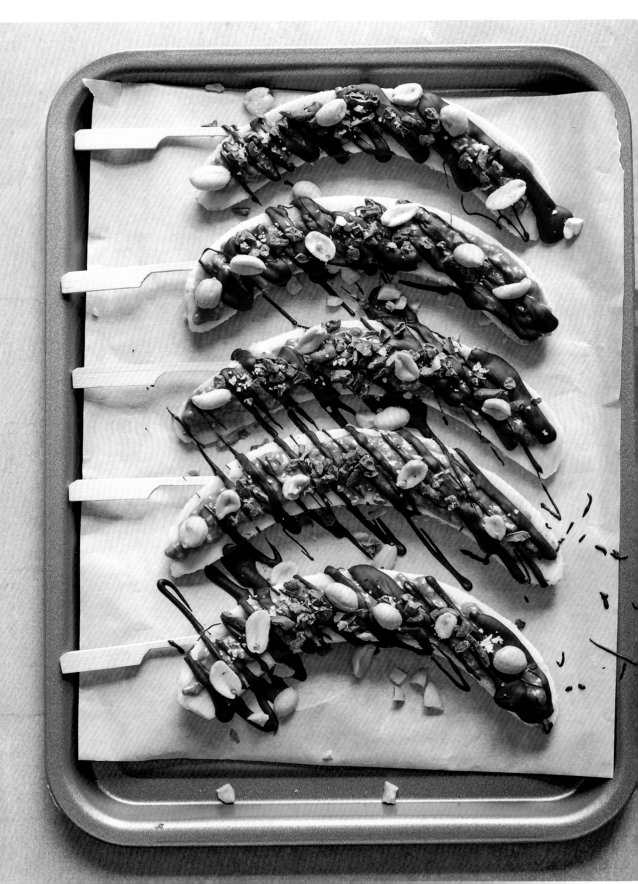

BANANA PEANUT POPSICLES

This is essentially a banana lollypop with added chocolate and nut butter, and it's a little bit of work but totally worth it.

Just find some yourself perfectly yellow bananas, which aren't too hard and aren't too soft. Fun fact: the most popular variety of banana is called the Cavendish!

Makes 6

3 medium yellow bananas

12 heaped teaspoons nut butter

100 g ($3\frac{1}{2}$ oz) 70 per cent chocolate

50 g (2 oz) cocoa nibs

50 g (2 oz) unsalted peanuts or almond nibs

sea salt flakes

Nutrition per serving:
Energy: 419 kcal | Total carbohydrate: 21 g (of which sugars: 16 g)
Fat: 30 g | Fibre: 6.6 g | Protein: 13 g | Salt: 0.35 g

1. Peel and cut your bananas in half lengthways, being careful not to break them.

2. Insert a wooden kebab-type skewer into the banana lengthways.

3. Line a tray with non-stick paper. Place the bananas on it and refrigerate.

4. Warm up the nut butter slightly to ensure it is soft. Remove the bananas from the fridge and spread the nut butter evenly along each half.

5. Freeze the bananas for 2–3 hours until they are frozen hard.

6. Melt the chocolate, take the bananas out of the freezer, and drizzle the chocolate over them, working quickly. Sprinkle the coco nibs, nuts and some sea salt flakes on top.

7. Place back in the freezer until you're ready to eat them. Any excess chocolate can be used in baking or eaten with a large spoon…

BEETROOT AND BUTTER BEAN HUMMUS WITH CRISPY BROAD BEANS

Based on habas fritas, the salty, roasted broad beans served as tapas, I first made this up while at a cycling training camp on the Spanish island of Majorca.

It's a smooth blend of nutritious ingredients topped with a crunch that goes really well with the slightly one-dimensional nature of the hummus. Spread on good quality crispy bread or fill a pitta for the road ahead.

Makes 6 servings

400 g (14 oz) butter beans, strained

200 g (7 oz) cooked beetroot

100 ml ($\frac{1}{2}$ cup) unsweetened beetroot juice

2 tablespoons white wine vinegar

190 ml olive oil (Spanish obviously)

salt and pepper

50 g (2 oz) crispy broad beans (also known as habas fritas)

Nutrition per serving:
Energy: 349 kcal | Total carbohydrate: 12 g (of which sugars: 5.3 g)
Fat: 30 g | Fibre: 5.3 g | Protein: 5.5 g | Salt: 0.09 g

1. Throw everything into a food processor with the exception of the broad beans. Blend.
2. Season then top with lots of the crispy broad beans.

Make a meal of it

Grilled chicken and a baked potato would work well. Or serve with ubiquitous vegetable crudités.

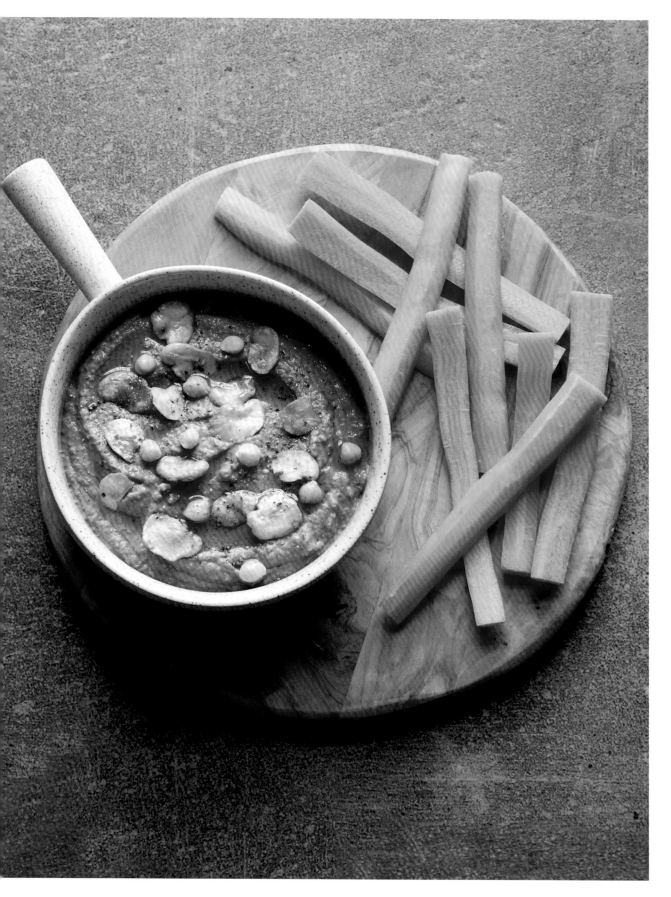

PRESSED PARMESAN AND ROSEMARY POLENTA

Fancy something a little different on the savoury side? Say hello to polenta! Rich in complex carbohydrates, it's arguably the most under-utilised carb in the portfolio.

These fritters are awesome as an on-the bike snack or as part of a hot savoury breakfast. The key to a successful fritter? Cook slowly and don't skimp on the Parmesan and black pepper.

Serves 4

150 g (5 oz) dry polenta

150 g (5 oz) semi-skimmed milk

450 ml (1¾ cups) chicken or vegetable stock or water

6 g rosemary, chopped

30 g (1¼ oz) unsalted butter

100 g (3½ oz) Parmesan cheese, grated

good grind of black pepper

olive oil

Nutrition per serving:

Energy: 344 kcal | Total carbohydrate: 30 g (of which sugars: 2.5 g)

Fat: 18 g | Fibre: 2.8 g | Protein: 14 g | Salt: 1.5 g

1. Line a 24 x 12 cm (2 lb) loaf tin.

2. Place the polenta in a heavy-bottomed pan. Add the milk, stock and rosemary.

3. Simmer for 8–10 minutes, stirring as you go, until it thickens up, which will take a few minutes.

4. Stir in the butter, cheese and pepper.

5. Pour it into the lined loaf tin and refrigerate overnight.

6. Cut the polenta into large chunks and sauté in the olive oil in a non-stick pan until golden brown.

7. If you're taking it on the bike, refrigerate before wrapping to firm it up again.

Make a meal of it

For breakfast, fried eggs and bacon or chicken/veggie sausages and baked beans.

JAM SOUFFLÉ BREAKFAST DESSERT

Dessert for breakfast? The decadent, fluffy soufflé omelette was trendy in haute cuisine back in the 1970s, but here it's rescued from the starched table cloth restaurant brigade for a protein-rich breakfast.

You could also consider replacing the jam with…. Nutella! Outrageous!

Serves 1

3 medium eggs

1 teaspoon whole milk

1 teaspoon sugar

3 teaspoons good quality jam

25 g (1 oz) unsalted butter

icing sugar

Nutrition per serving:
Energy: 622 kcal | Total carbohydrate: 52 g (of which sugars: 49 g)
Fat: 36 g | Fibre: 0 g | Protein: 22 g | Salt: 0.67 g

1. Preheat the oven to 190°C/375°F/Gas 5.
2. Separate the eggs. In one bowl mix together the yolks, milk, sugar and 1 teaspoon of the jam, reserving the rest.
3. Whisk the egg whites until they form soft peaks.
4. Take a third of your egg whites and mix with the egg yolks. Then fold this back into the remaining whites.
5. Heat the butter in a large non-stick ovenproof pan over a medium to high heat. When it's sizzling pour in the egg mix and cook for 1 minute.
6. Place the pan in the oven for 4–5 minutes until the soufflé puffs up.
7. Remove from the oven. Be careful – the pan handle will be very hot!
8. Turn the soufflé on to a plate, spoon on some more jam and dust with icing sugar.

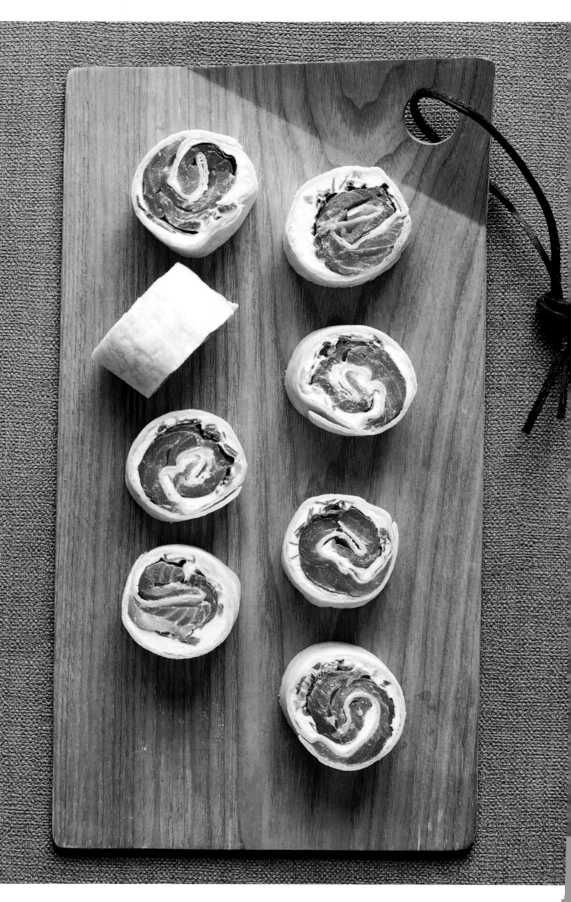

SMOKED SALMON AND CREAM CHEESE ROULADE

Smoked salmon and cream cheese is a classic combination and with good reason.

Throw in some baby spinach leaves and you're away. Don't be put-off by the roulade business – it's just a matter of rolling the tortilla wrap. The point is that this is much easier to handle on the bike than, say, a bagel would be.

Serves 2

2 large tortilla wraps

2 tablespoons full fat cream cheese

4 spring onions, chopped

handful baby spinach leaves

120 g (4 oz) sliced smoked salmon

1. Take the wraps and spread them with cream cheese.
2. Sprinkle on the spring onions.
3. Lay out a layer of spinach leaves.
4. Next add a layer of salmon.
5. Roll up and refrigerate to set.
6. Cut and wrap bite-sized pieces for easy consumption.

Nutrition per serving:

Energy: 381 kcal | Total carbohydrate: 34 g (of which sugars: 2.5 g)

Fat: 17 g | Fibre: 2.4 g | Protein: 21 g | Salt: 3.1 g

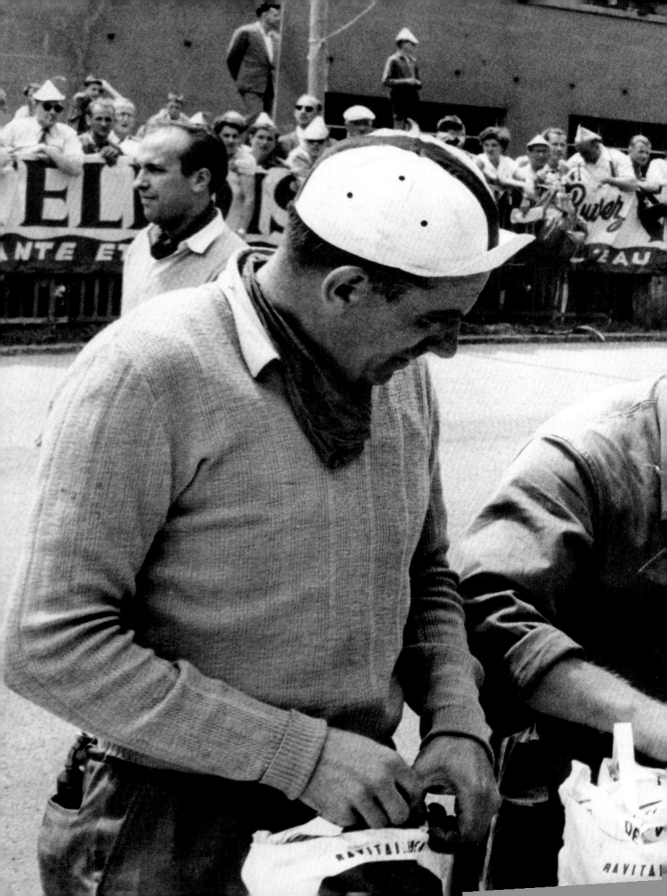

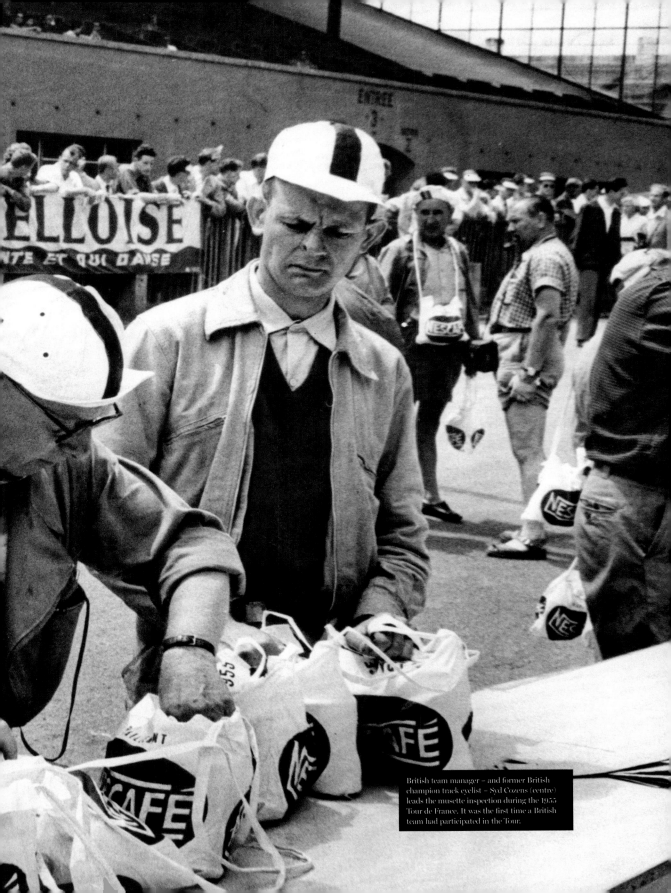

British team manager – and former British champion track cyclist – Syd Cozens (centre) leads the musette inspection during the 1955 Tour de France. It was the first time a British team had participated in the Tour.

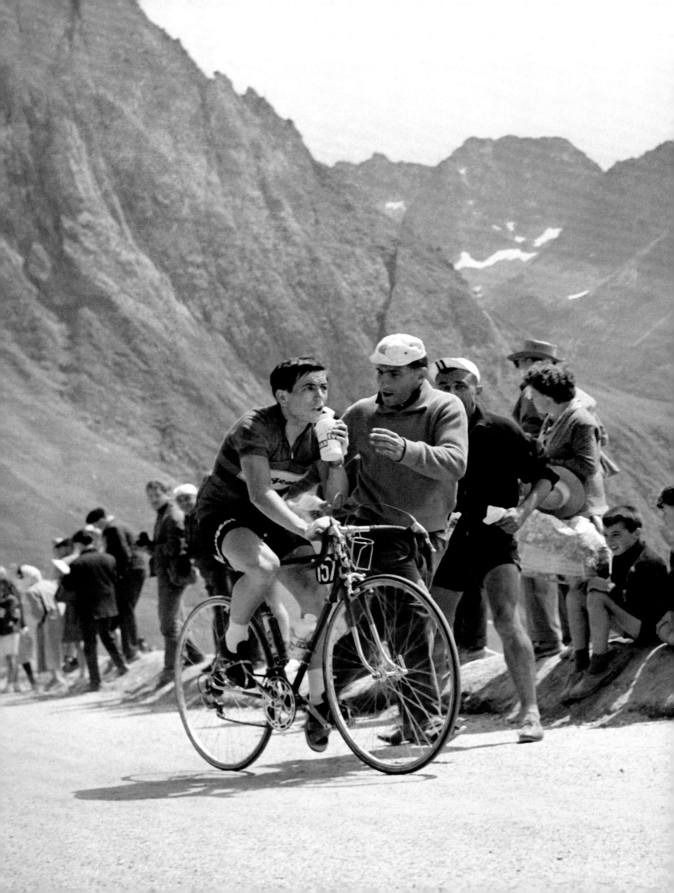

OPTIMUM HYDRATION

Adult men's bodies are around 60 per cent water, women are nearer 55 per cent. Either way, that's a lot of water and we can learn two things straight away: first, water is pretty vital to our health; second, we can afford to lose a little without serious consequences. Both of these are relevant to how much we need to hydrate while on the bike. Just like our carbohydrate intake, assuming our tank is full before we set off we then need to ensure we are adequately topping it up throughout the ride.

Thirsty work as a rider in the 1960 Tour de France tackles the dramatic and intimidating col du Tourmalet. The mountain in the Pyrenees has been used more often in the Tour de France than any other climb.

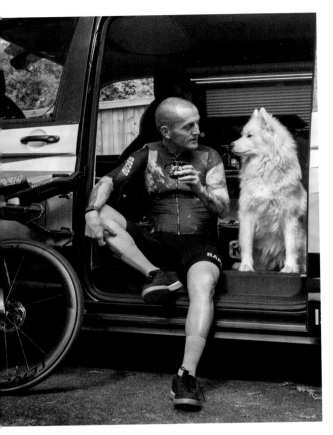

Post-ride analysis with a seriously unimpressed Farley.

The water in our bodies is vital to our performance levels. It lubricates our muscles, tissues and joints, enables us to sweat and disperse heat, and facilitates blood flow to muscles and organs, including the heart, the digestive system and the brain. Levels of hydration can affect stamina, fatigue, aerobic capacity and concentration. You'll find dehydration calculated by a percentage of body weight with negative effects beginning at 2 per cent dehydration. At that level most cyclists won't notice any significant consequences, but at around 3 per cent dehydration it can have an impact on muscular performance, and by 5 per cent you might feel some of the effects of heat exhaustion.

Fortunately, there is an easy way to calculate your dehydration level after riding. Weigh yourself (in minimal clothing) as near as possible to the start and then again at the finish of your ride. The difference in your weight (adding any fluid taken on during the ride) is almost all water. One litre of sweat will weigh 1 kg. For an 80 kg rider this means a 0.8 kg weight reduction is 1 per cent, a 2.4 kg drop is 3 per cent and a 4 kg reduction accounts for 5 per cent dehydration. A more ad hoc method is to check the colour of your urine. A well-hydrated body produces clear to slightly yellow urine, whereas a deeper yellow or amber colour indicates increasing levels of dehydration.

SWEATING THE SMALL STUFF

Sweating is a pretty efficient cooling system – well, it beats panting like a dog. When we over-heat, the sweat glands from our head to our toes (mostly concentrated on the palms, soles, forehead, armpits, groin and breasts) produce moisture which is converted to vapour using that excess body heat. The downside is that sweating releases vital water from the body and, although it is mainly water, sweat also contains protein waste products such as urea and ammonia, but more importantly electrolytes, including potassium and sodium.

A potassium deficit can lead to muscle weakness, but the amount lost by sweating has a pretty negligible effect. Sports drink packaging usually implies that you need to replace those losses immediately, but the urgency tends to be overstated. A litre of sweat will contain only around 2.5 per cent of the recommended daily intake of potassium. A small potato, banana or an electrolyte drink will easily replace the potassium you lose in a couple of hours of intense riding, and only if you habitually sweat very heavily and have a diet low in potassium might it cause any serious issues.

Sodium is an altogether different proposition, though. This is the salt you lose in your sweat, and you need it. How much is lost varies enormously from person to person and can be as low as 200 mg or over 2000 mg per litre. That means some riders lose the recommended daily intake of sodium (1500 mg) in an hour or so and most will lose that over the course of a hard ride. Sodium is vital to regulate the balance of fluid in the body and to maintain normal blood pressure. It helps the absorption of nutrients in the gut, and is also integral to the contraction and relaxation of muscles (although the links with cramp are disputed by some). In other words, it's pretty important.

Unlike sweating there are no easy ways to measure your sodium levels, although there are some tell-tale signs that the rate at which you lose salt is high. For instance, you might discover white rings or salt stains on your clothes after a ride; you might find your sweat stings your eyes or tastes salty; or maybe the dog seems to find licking your arms and legs especially appealing. If you're a salty rider, it's usually down to genetics, but can also be affected by how much salt you generally have in your diet. Specialist companies do provide sweat

A litre of sweat will contain only around 2.5 per cent of the recommended daily intake of potassium. A small potato, banana or an electrolyte drink will easily replace the potassium you lose in a couple of hours of intense riding.

testing to assess sodium levels and might be worth investing in if you have concerns. Your rate will not change significantly, so one test will suffice.

Although piling – or should that be shaking or grinding – on the salt isn't considered good in your everyday diet, just like sugar, it is the opposite when you're on the bike. Salt is an essential part of your on-ride fuelling. Every time you drink without taking on any extra salt you are diluting the sodium level in your blood. This can become a problem if you're a heavy sweater and excessively drink just water – through over-zealousness, over a long ride of more than five hours or in high humidity or heat. You might experience nausea, headaches or lethargy, which could lead to more serious issues. However, you can easily avoid this by eating something salty or by adding a little salt to your water. However, don't rely on sports drinks without checking the ingredients as some provide insufficient sodium. As a rule of thumb, try to take on around half a teaspoon of salt for every litre of fluid lost through sweat.

It is clear that we need to keep our bodies hydrated and our electrolyte levels stable. How much we sweat is down to the intensity of the ride and the weather, the fitness of the rider (the fitter you are the more efficient your body is at cooling itself) and the individual sweat rate of the rider. We need to replace some of the fluid lost, but not necessarily all. It is impossible for Grand Tour riders climbing in high temperatures to imbibe enough fluids to replace all their losses and yet their performance is not affected.

As every rider will have different fluid levels, it would be foolhardy for me to tell you how much to drink. You need to be sensitive to your own body's requirements and how it reacts in different situations. This can be fine-tuned in training rides and assessed by using the previously described weight test.

However, as a start, there are some basic guidelines. Unless it is a particularly hot day or an intense ride, you don't need any specific pre-ride plan or to drink extra prior to the start of the race. Just ensure that you're continually hydrated in the 24 hours beforehand. On the bike, begin with the old adage, drink to thirst. If your mouth feels dry take a couple of gulps of water. You might only take a couple of sips in the first hour as your body will already have reserves of a couple of litres. As the ride continues, take a gulp every 15 minutes, so you're getting through about half to three-quarters of a bidon in an hour. If you feel hot, thirsty or sweaty (remember most of your sweat will evaporate without you noticing) then increase your fluid intake.

After the ride, re-hydration should be an integral part of your recovery programme. Over the next day you should be looking to replace all the lost fluid on top of your normal intake. Unless you have sweated substantially or have another ride that day, it is fine to take your time and rehydrate alongside replenishing electrolytes, carbohydrates and protein. With a healthy diet there is no real need for a specific sports drink, but drinking water with meals will help water retention.

Much of this is instinct and common sense. You need to keep hydrated, but generally regular small amounts of water will be enough. In average conditions and moderate riding expect to get through a couple of bidons on a three-hour ride, but make sure you have some form of sodium, whether it is in the drink or in food. I have to stress, though, that hydration is unique to every individual and it's important enough to spend time and effort in training to identify the right solutions for you.

BASIC ISOTONIC DRINK RECIPE

Many sports drinks try to provide a one-stop shop for the fluid, electrolytes and energy you lose through exercise. However, not only are they expensive, but they can also be highly processed and may contain preservatives, artificial flavourings and sweeteners or high amounts of sugar that can distort your carbohydrate intake.

Coconut water has also been marketed as a natural alternative, but it is not a viable option, because, although it has high levels of potassium, it has insufficient sodium to replace what you lose when sweating reasonably heavily.

Making your own isotonic drink is dead easy and can be made to your personal requirements. All you need to do is fill a bidon three-quarters full with tap water. Top it up with fruit juice, add one tablespoon of table sugar and half a teaspoon of salt then give it a good shake.

The inclusion of salt and sugar increases the speed at which the water is absorbed into your bloodstream, but adjust the level of sweetness and saltiness to suit your requirements. It will be most effective if you use apple, pomegranate, grape or another high fructose juice, but it's more important to choose something you will enjoy drinking.

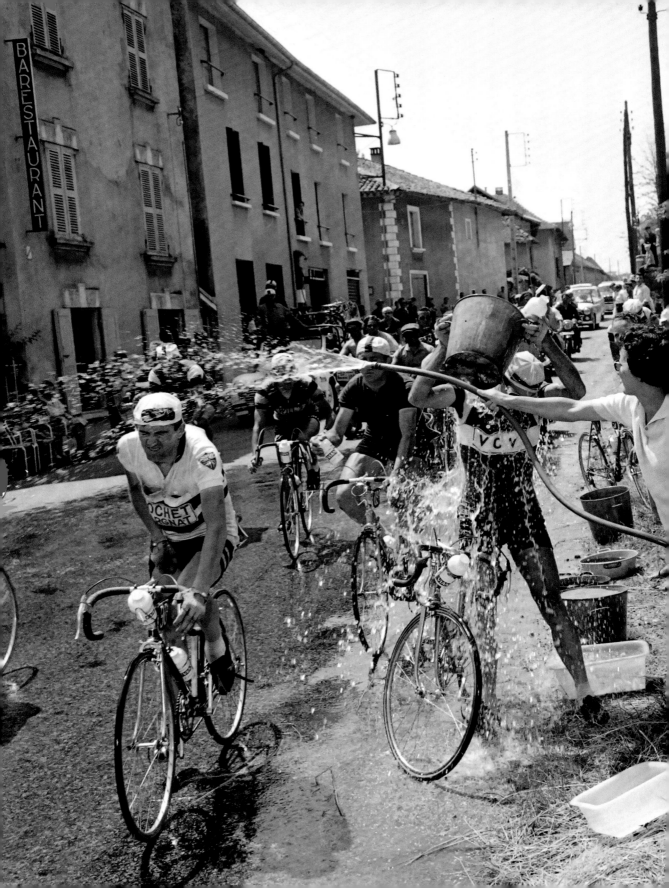

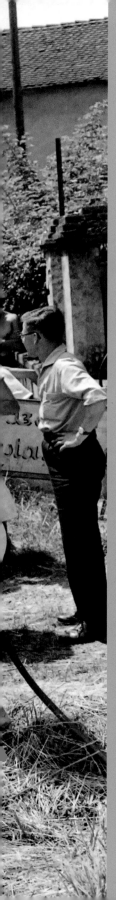

RECIPES

WORKING UP A THIRST

We've seen how vital hydration is to both
our wellbeing and our performance on
the bike, but thankfully liquid lubrication
is welcome no matter how exhausted
you feel. Whether it's Liquorice, lemon
and lime drink (see page 178), a hearty
protein- and carbo-heavy soup like
Chowder for the road (see page 184) or
a comforting Silky smooth hot chocolate
(see page 181), a drop of the wet stuff is
just the ticket.

Cyclists using every possible
way to cool down during the
ninth stage of the 1961 Tour
de France between Saint-
Etienne and Grenoble.

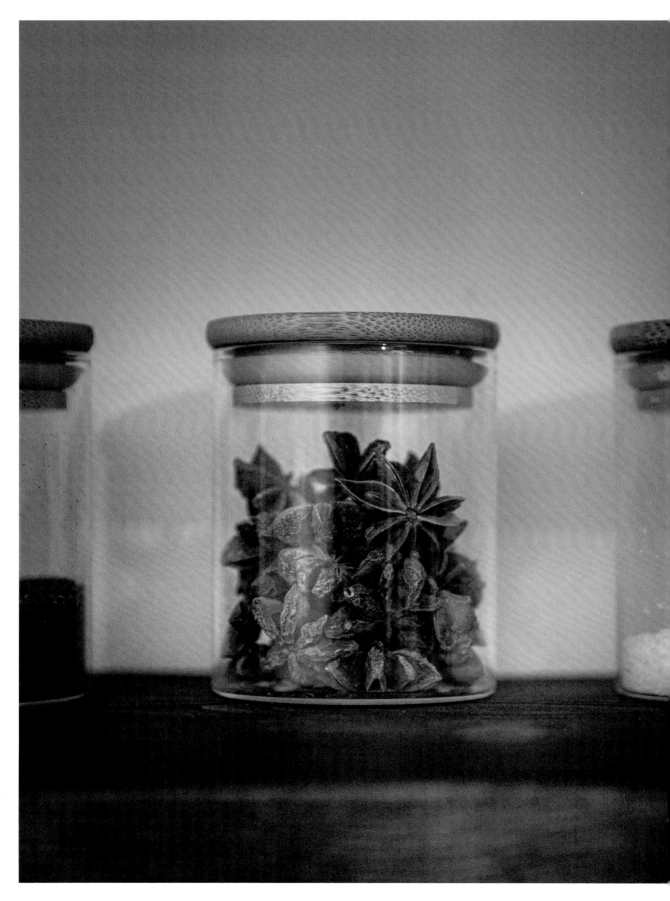

SPICY CYCLISTS' CHAI

Chai is essentially a hot, spiced, sweet tea, because – trust me – on cold wet days the last thing you want is a cold drink.

Invest in an insulated bike bottle as the morale boost you get from a hot cuppa when things getting grippy cannot be underestimated. What's even better is that each couple of cups provides about the same amount of carbs as those fancy expensive energy drinks! The recipe below makes 6 servings of the dry ingredients so they can be stored in advance, making this delicious drink really simple to make.

Dry ingredients, makes 6 servings

50 g (2 oz) cassia cinnamon bark (from Asian supermarkets)

5 star anise

10 cardamom pods

6 whole cloves

4 black peppercorns

80 g (3 oz) crystallised ginger

1 teaspoon dried ginger powder

50 g (2 oz) loose black tea (I like Assam)

20 g ($\frac{3}{4}$ oz) Sencha green tea leaves, vanilla if you can get them

Liquid ingredients per serving

200 ml ($\frac{3}{4}$ cup) boiling water

100 ml ($\frac{1}{2}$ cup) sweetened condensed milk

50 ml (3 tablespoons) sweetened almond milk

Nutrition per serving:
Energy (Kcal): 341 Kcal | Fat: 9 g | Carbohydrate: 59 g
(of which sugars): 58 g | Fibre: 0 g | Protein: 7 g | Salt: 0.2 g

1. Start by lightly crushing all the dry ingredients in the food processor.

2. Put one serving – 33 g ($1\frac{1}{4}$ oz) – of the dry mix in a jug. Add 400 ml ($1\frac{1}{2}$ cups) boiling water, 100 g ($\frac{1}{2}$ cup) condensed milk (less if you prefer it not to be too sweet) and 50 ml almond milk.

3. Allow to infuse for 5–6 minutes.

4. Strain through a fine sieve into a pan and reheat the chai. Then pour it into a preheated insulated cycling bidon or flask.

5. Store the rest of the mix in an airtight container for another time.

Old favourites, forgotten flavours and newly discovered delights: the spice shelf is a thing of beauty and inspiration.

LIQUORICE, LEMON AND LIME ENERGY DRINK

The legendary Beryl Burton famously snacked on liquorice allsorts during her time trial wins. Here that liquorice fuel source is brought up to date and turned into a drink.

Less sweet than the usual carb drinks, the liquorice, citrus juice and salt create an altogether more balanced flavour profile in tribute to one of Britain's best. Once you've made the syrup base, keep the liquorice to eat as ride food, BB style.

Makes 2 servings

80 g (3 oz) white sugar

50 g (2 oz) black liquorice

80 g (3 oz) lemon juice

20 g ($\frac{3}{4}$ oz) lime juice

1 teaspoon Himalayan pink salt

200 ml ($\frac{3}{4}$ cup) water

500 ml (2 cups) sparkling water (or more if you want fewer carbs in your drink)

Nutrition per serving:

Energy: 244 kcal | Total carbohydrate: 56 g (of which sugars: 51 g)
Fat: 0.5 g | Fibre: 0.5 g | Protein: 1.5 g | Salt: 2.1 g

1. Place all the ingredients apart from sparkling water in a saucepan and reduce over a medium or high heat until you have a syrup. The ideal weight to have left is 170 g (6 oz) including the chunks of liquorice.

2. Pour into a jug, cool and refrigerate, ideally leaving it overnight to infuse.

3. When you're ready to use, add ice cold sparkling water.

4. If you like this mix you can obviously make up a big batch as it keeps forever in the fridge.

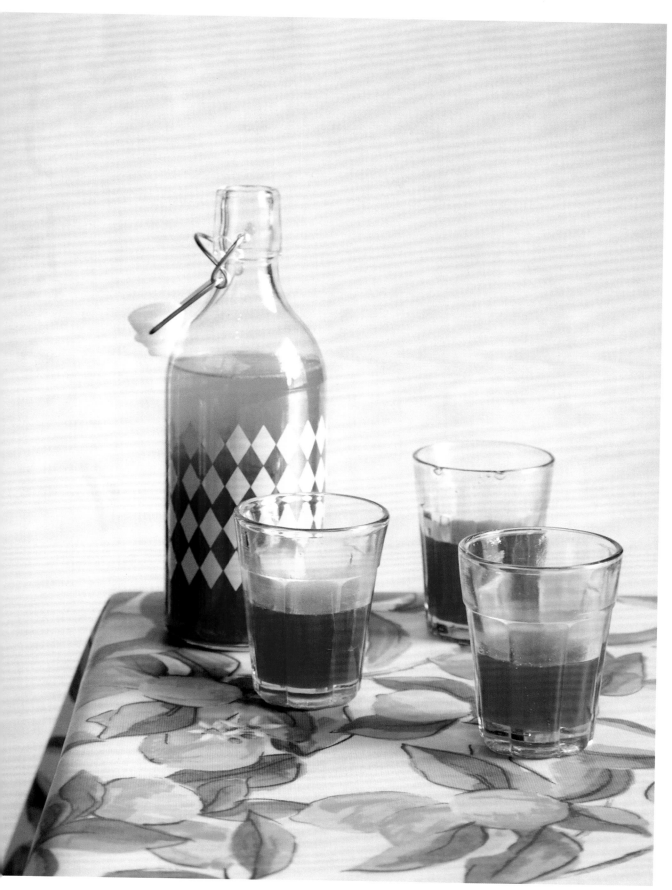

STIGGY SMOOTHIE

Red rocket fuel! Beetroot juice, spinach, banana… there's absolutely nothing here that's not going to put a tiger in the tank…

This is a pre-race beet smoothie favoured by multiple world champion, mountain biker Laura Stigger. Keep a batch in the fridge for a daily morning blast and remember to give it a good shake before serving.

Serves 3

400 ml (1½ cups) beetroot juice

400 ml (1½ cups) apple juice

300 g (11 oz) mixed frozen berries

160 g (5½ oz) full fat Greek yoghurt

100 g (3½ oz) baby spinach leaves

1 large banana

1. Blend all the ingredients together.
2. Store in the fridge in 500 ml (2 cups) bottles for the three days prior to your big ride out.

Nutrition per serving:
Energy: 245 kcal | Total carbohydrate: 41 g (of which sugars: 38 g)
Fat: 4.3 g | Fibre: 4 g | Protein: 8.5 g | Salt: 0.29 g

SILKY SMOOTH HOT CHOCOLATE

Hot chocolate and cycling go back a long, long way. Apparently, the 1904 Tour de France winner Henri Cornet drank 11 litres of hot chocolate during his successful campaign!

I doubt very much he had anything as decadent as this gently spiced, luxury hot chocolate – with protein powder and marshmallows! Recovery has never ever tasted so good.

Serves 2

1 tablespoon brown sugar

650 ml (2¾ cups) whole milk

50 g (2 oz) unsweetened cocoa powder

pinch of cinnamon

pinch of allspice

100 g (3½ oz) chocolate protein powder

100 g (3½ oz) full fat Greek yoghurt

70 g (3 oz) marshmallows

Nutrition per serving:

Energy: 704 kcal | Total carbohydrate: 59 g (of which sugars: 50 g)

Fat: 23 g | Fibre: 3.4 g | Protein: 64 g | Salt: 0.95 g

1. Sprinkle the sugar into a pan and gently heat until it has melted and formed a sugary base on the bottom of the pan. This ensures the milk does not stick to the bottom of the pan (it's a top cheffy tip and you can thank me later).

2. Add the milk, cocoa powder, cinnamon and allspice, and bring gently to a light simmer.

3. Remove from the heat and pour into a blender. On low, speed add the protein powder, yoghurt and marshmallows. Then give it a quick blast until it's silky.

4. Return the chocolate mix to the pan, heat gently to bring back up to temperature, pour into two mugs, add a dust of coco powder if you like and enjoy.

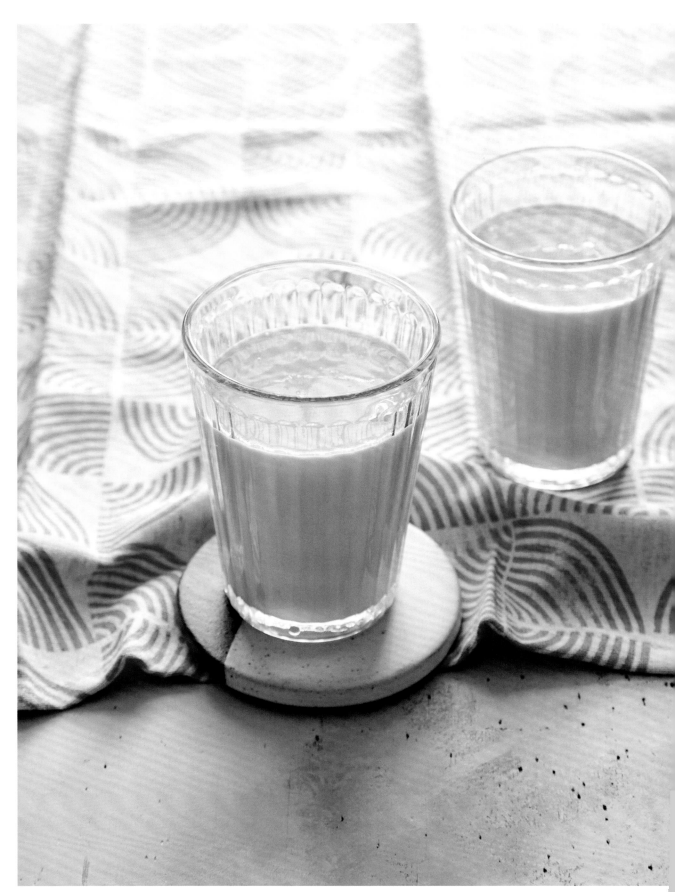

FULL-GAS LASSI

The perfect pre-ride bang-for-your-buck breakfast in a glass.

Mango, coconut and yoghurt combine in a refreshing and energising tropical-style smoothie to set you on your way. If the day is particularly full-on then switch up the coconut milk to the full fat variety for more calories minus the bulk.

Serves 2

200 g (7 oz) frozen mango

200 ml ($\frac{3}{4}$ cup) light coconut milk

200 ml ($\frac{3}{4}$ cup) unsweetened oat or almond milk

100 g ($3\frac{1}{2}$ oz) full fat Greek yoghurt

1 teaspoon honey or maple syrup

pinch of turmeric powder

pinch of ground cardamom

handful of ice

1. Blend all the ingredients together until smooth.

2. Pour into a glass and drink.

Nutrition per serving:
Energy: 249 kcal | Total carbohydrate: 25 g (of which sugars: 22 g)
Fat: 13 g | Fibre: 2.9 g | Protein: 7.3 g | Salt: 0.24 g

CHOWDER FOR THE ROAD

When the cold wind bites reach for the chowder as protein and carbs come together here in one deliciously warming rich, thick, smoky, fishy soup.

There is always a place for carbs without the sweetness and a chowder is just the ticket. Obviously, you need an insulated bottle or flask to take this on the road.

Serves 6

75 ml (4½ tablespoons) olive oil

75 g (3 oz) butter

1 large onion, finely chopped

1 stick celery, finely chopped

400 g (14 oz) smoked haddock

2 teaspoons turmeric

1 tablespoon mild curry powder

240 g (9 oz) sweetcorn

800 g (1 lb 7 oz) potato, diced

350 ml (1½ cups) semi-skimmed milk

500 ml (2 cups) chicken stock

salt and pepper

1. Melt the oil and butter in a pan. Add the onion and celery, and cook for 4–5 minutes until they have a little colour.
2. Add the smoked haddock, turmeric and curry powder. Cook for a further 3–4 minutes.
3. Add the sweetcorn, potato, milk and stock.
4. Simmer for 20-25 minutes, ensuring the chowder doesn't stick to the bottom of the pan.
5. Remove from the heat and allow to cool for 45 minutes.
6. Blend until smooth, add a touch more stock if it's too thick and season.
7. Reheat as required.

Nutrition per serving:

Energy: 464 kcal | Total carbohydrate: 36 g (of which sugars: 9.4 g)
Fat: 25 g | Fibre: 5.3 g | Protein: 21 g | Salt: 1.1 g

GET ME HOME LENTIL SOUP

Here is a hearty and comforting soup to stoke you for that final hour of a ride or warm your bones when you get home.

When I was growing up, this is the sort of soup – without the harissa – that would always be on the hob and it's best made a day in advance, but take care not to end up with a big pan of mush.

Serves 6

2 tablespoons olive oil

60 g (2½ oz) unsalted butter

1 kg (2¼ lb) veg, diced – for example, carrot, sweet potato, celery and onion

180 g (6 oz) smoked back bacon, diced

1 tablespoon harissa paste

300 g (11 oz) red lentils

2000 ml (4 pints) chicken stock

Nutrition per serving:

Energy: 422 kcal | Total carbohydrate: 50 g (of which sugars: 13 g)
Fat: 15 g | Fibre: 7.3 g | Protein: 19 g | Salt: 2.4 g

1. Melt the oil and butter in a pan. Add the veg and cook over a medium heat for 8–10 minutes.

2. Add the bacon and harissa, and cook for a further 5 minutes.

3. Add the lentils and stock. Simmer for 30 minutes, then turn off the heat and allow to sit a while with the lid on.

4. When it's cool, blend and adjust the seasoning.

5. Reheat as required.

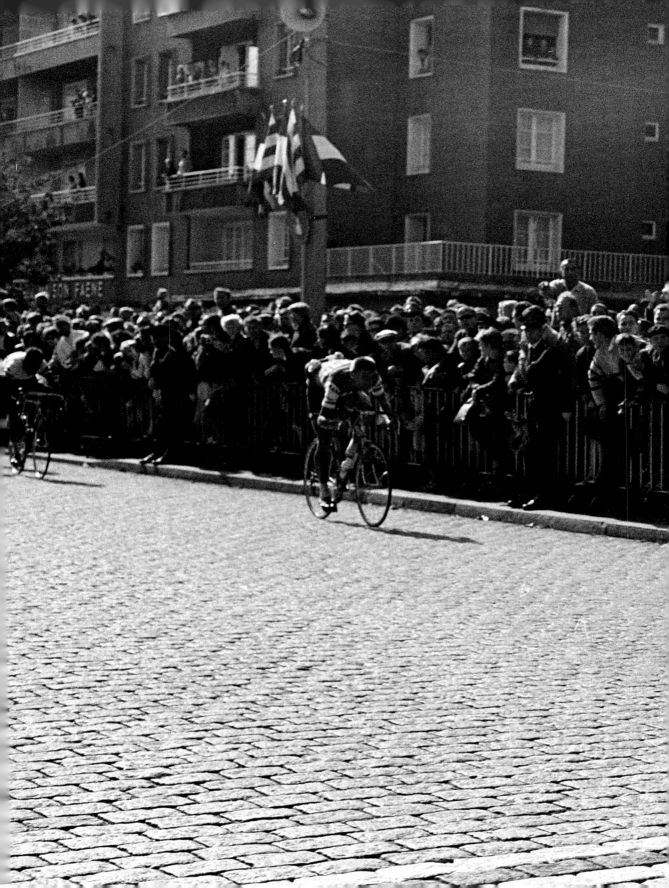